THE COMPLETE GUIDE TO
RUBBERIZED RESISTANCE EXERCISES

THE COMPLETE GUIDE TO

RUBBERIZED RESISTANCE EXERCISES

Written by: MARK CIBRARIO, C.S.C.S.

Consultants: MARK STONE, BS
& CONNIE LOVE, MA

Models: MARK CIBRARIO
TRACY CAMPANELLA
& KAREN REDMOND

By: **SPRI PRODUCTS, INC.**

MUNDELEIN, ILLINOIS 60060

1.5M2000

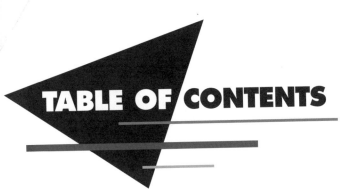

TABLE OF CONTENTS

GENERAL GUIDELINES

1. Select appropriate rubberized resistance based on your strength level. If moderate to maximum muscle fatigue is not reached by your predetermined repetition goal, choose a heavier resistance. If you are unable to complete a minimum of eight repetitions, choose a lighter resistance. Each exercise may require a different color band or length of rubberized resistance (see loading resistance progression).

2. Before starting an exercise, move away from the tubing insertion to a point where the level of tension is constant throughout the entire range of motion. There should be no excessive slack from the hand to the insertion. The pre-stretch applied to the rubber can increase resistance, but do not allow the rubber to stretch beyond three times its resting length at any time.

3. Always control the resistance, especially during the return phase of the movement. The recommended eccentric phase should be 2 to 4 seconds. This rule should be remembered with the phrase: "You control the resistance tool, it doesn't control you".

4. If any discomfort or excessive strain is felt at the musculo-tendonous junction, near any joint, move body toward attachment site to reduce tension or choose a lighter resistance.

5. Perform an equal number of repetitions with each arm or leg and work opposing muscle groups equally to avoid muscular imbalances.

6. Before each use, always inspect the rubberized resistance for nicks and tears that may occur from continued use. Avoid prolonged exposure to sunlight, salt, or chlorine treated water.

7. Never tie any two pieces of rubber together.

8. Perform each exercise as described.

9. Consult your physician before beginning any type of exercise program.

TUBING ANCHORING GUIDELINES:

** When anchoring tubing with a door strap, make sure it is securely attached prior to performing the exercise by giving tubing a firm tug.

Listed below are optional ways to anchor tubing:

1. Around feet (See page 7)
2. In door jam (Xergym doorstrap) (See page 9)
3. Around immovable objects i.e. pole, weight machine, beam (double loop doorstrap) (See page 10)
4. Tubing nook i.e. board with o-rings spaced every two inches. (double loop doorstrap) (See page 11)
5. To step block (See pages 12 & 13)

XERCISE BAR/XERTUBE STANCE GUIDELINES

Unless a specific foot position is noted when standing on tubing, follow this progression before moving to the next level of resistance (See page 6)

BEGINNER   Place the middle of tubing under the arch of front or rear foot. Stand in a narrow staggered lunge stance.

INTERMEDIATE   Place the tubing evenly under the arches of both feet. Stand in a narrow square stance (feet hip width apart or slightly inside).

ADVANCED   Place the tubing evenly under the arches of both feet. Stand in a wide square stance (feet just outside hip width).

BODY ALIGNMENT GUIDELINES

For exercises performed seated or standing:

- Keep torso upright
- Head and neck in a neutral position
- Bellybutton drawn toward spine to avoid excessive arching of the low back and to provide spinal stabilization
- Eyes focused straight ahead

XERTUBE

XERTUBE™ RESISTANCE CHART

COLOR	RESISTANCE
YELLOW	BEGINNER
GREEN	BEGINNER/INTERMEDIATE
RED	INTERMEDIATE/ADVANCED
BLUE	ADVANCED
BLACK	VERY ADVANCED

STANCES

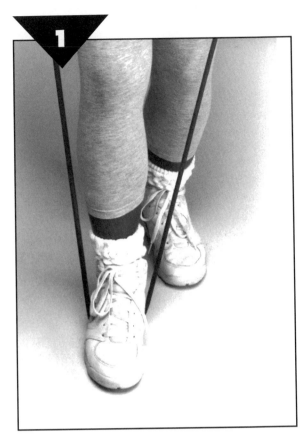

Staggered Narrow Stance

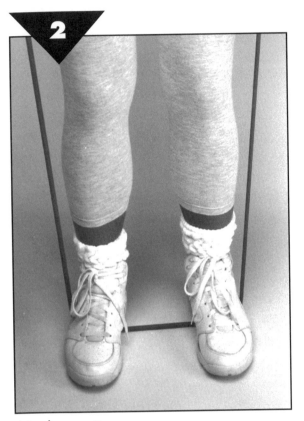

Moderate Stance

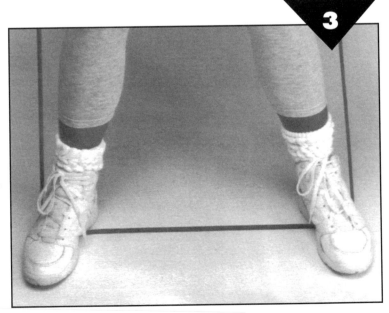

Wide Stance

FOOT WRAP

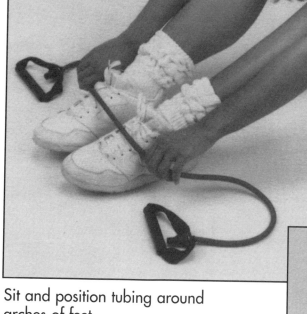

Sit and position tubing around arches of feet.

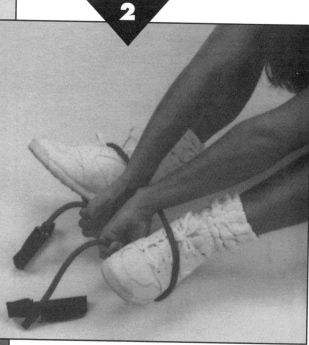

Cross tubing securely over the top of feet and under the instep/arches of your feet.

Grasp handles. Position feet together, bend knees, place feet on floor.

STRAP ATTACHMENT TO TUBING

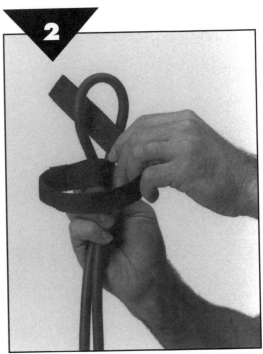

Feed other end of strap through opening.

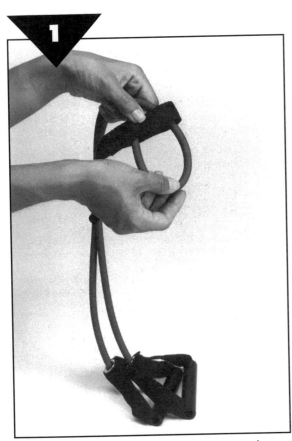

Fold tubing in half and grasp near end as shown. Place small loop of strap over end and leave space for other end of strap to fit through (same for Xergym Door Strap and double loop strap).

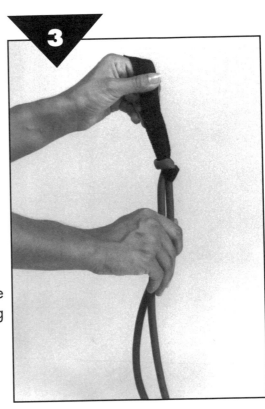

Pull tight to assure secure anchoring

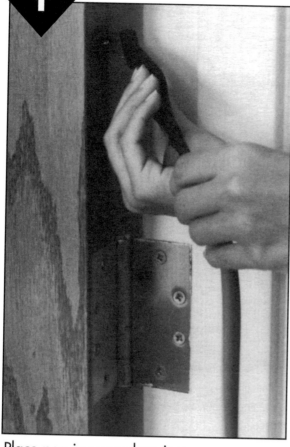

Place peg in open door jam.

DOOR JAM

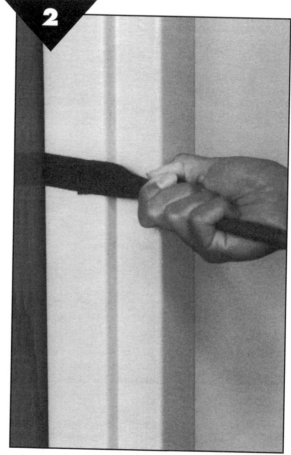

Close door with peg on inside. Tug to assure a safe anchoring.

ANCHORING TUBING TO A POLE OR MACHINE

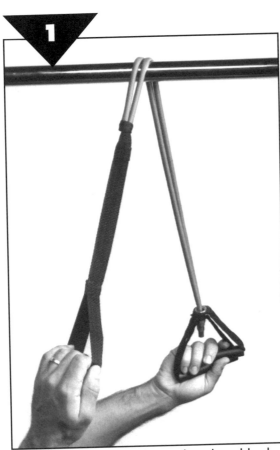

Grasp open loop with one hand and both handles with the other. Place around pole or beam as shown.

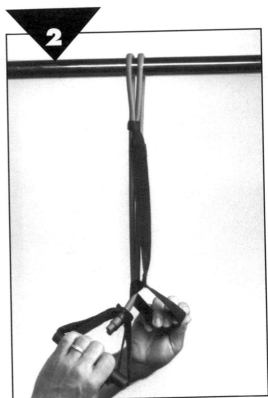

Feed handles through open loop.

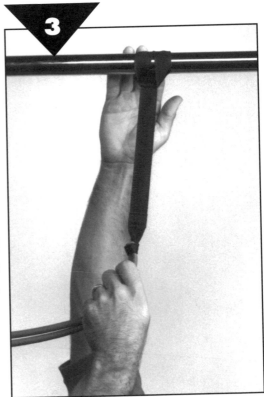

Pull handles through and tighten. Tug to assure secure anchoring.

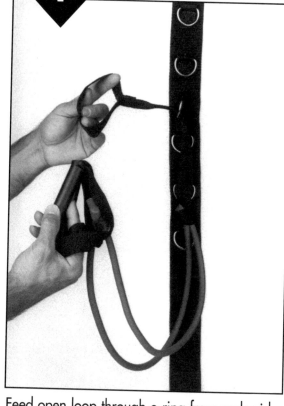

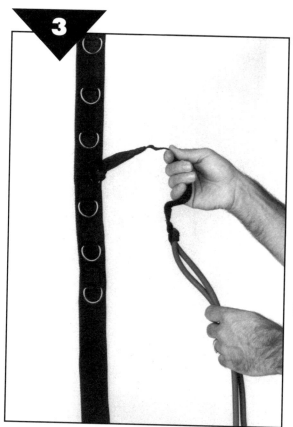

Feed open loop through o-ring from underside

Feed handles through loop.

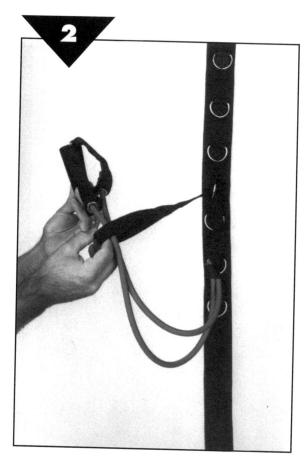

Pull tight to assure a secure anchoring.

STEP STRAP

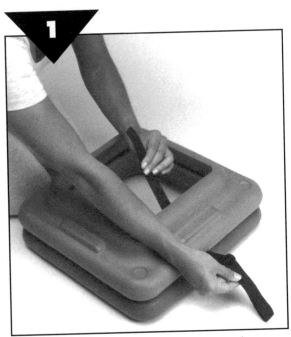

Place strap underneath one block with top of buckle facing up.

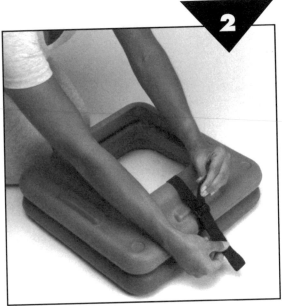

Pull long piece of strap over the block…

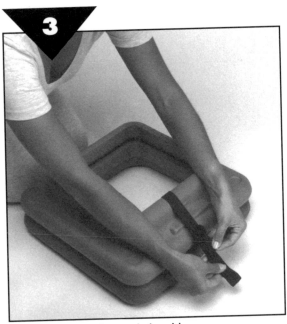

…and secure through buckle.

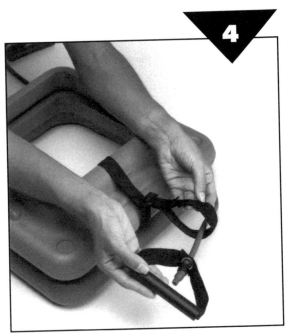

Slide one handle of the tube through the loop until step strap is in the middle of the tubing.

INSIDE-OUTSIDE STEP ATTACHMENTS

STEP STRAP ATTACHMENTS

For all exercises performed on the step, strap is secured around an adjustable step block, either inside or outside the attachment.

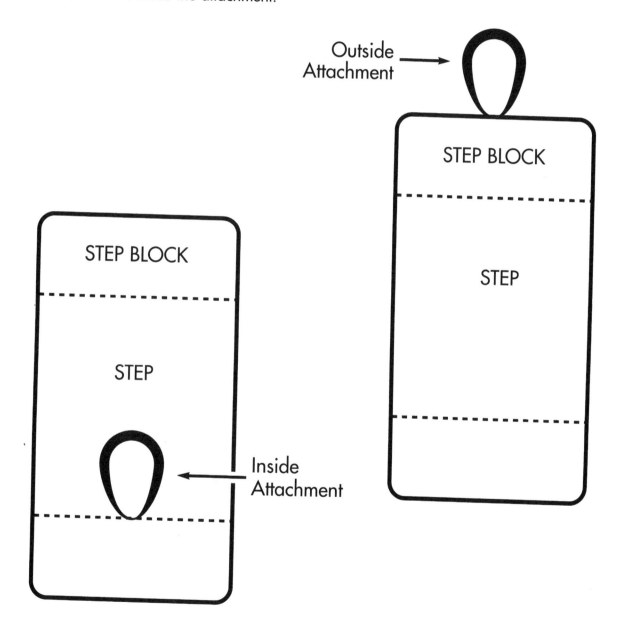

Outside Attachment →

STEP BLOCK

STEP

STEP BLOCK

STEP

← Inside Attachment

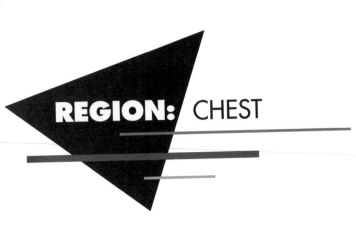

XERTUBE STANDING SINGLE ARM CHEST PRESS
(Pectorals)

A. Anchor tubing at lower chest height when standing. Face away from attachment site and align tubing slightly outside shoulder of exercising arm.

B. Move away from attachment site to desired tension level and assume a staggered lunge stance with leg opposite the exercising arm forward. Keep knees bent slightly, hips back, pelvis tilted slightly anterior, lumbar spine neutral, and lean torso forward slightly. Grasp handle(s) in hand with thumb up and positioned parallel to lower chest (low position) with shoulder abducted approximately 30° or position the hand with palm down, parallel to lower chest (high position) with shoulder abducted approximately 70°.

C. Extend the opposite arm fully at chest height in a punch-out position. Keep the spine in its neutral position, but allow the torso to turn slightly away from midline on the tubing side.

D. Press out and up with the resisted arm fully in the low or high plane of motion while bending the opposite arm, driving the elbow back. The torso should turn in the opposite motion as in the starting position. The eyes should focus in front of the foot of the lead leg. The starting lunge stance must be maintained, but the hip of the back leg should naturally rotate inward while the heel lifts slightly. The rib cage should be lifted high, lumbar curvature neutral (not rounded), and bellybutton drawn toward spine.

E. Slowly return to the starting position. Move the body so that the opposite arm is positioned correctly and repeat an equal amount of repetitions.

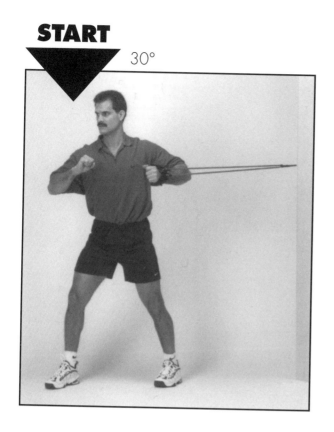

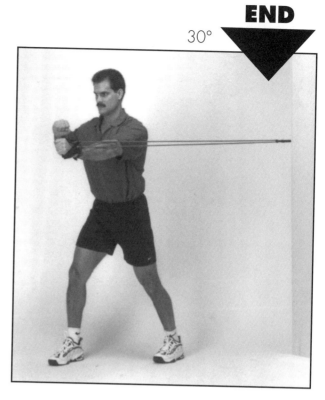

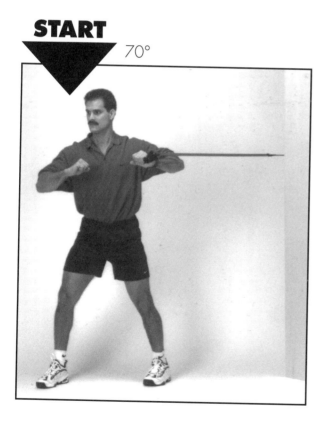

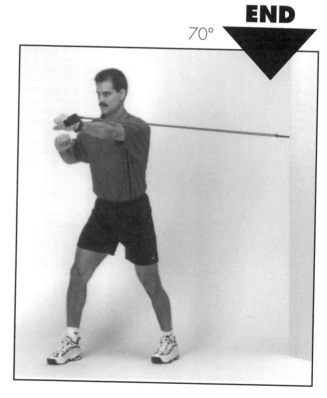

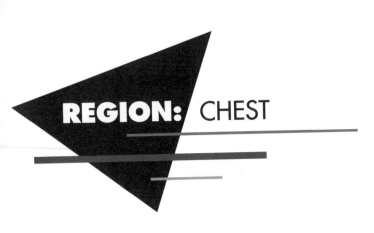

REGION: CHEST

XERTUBE PARTNER STANDING SINGLE ARM CHEST PRESS

(Pectorals)

A. Exerciser stands back-to-back with partner and each person grasps one handle with the same hand.

**For greater tension use two Xertubes.

B. Move away from each other taking steps forward to a desired tension level and assume a staggered lunge stance with the leg opposite the exercising arm forward. Keep knees bent slightly, hips back, pelvis tilted slightly anterior, lumbar spine neutral, and lean torso forward slightly. Position the hand with thumb up and parallel to lower chest (low position) with shoulder abducted approximately 30° or position the hand with palm down, parallel to lower chest (high position) with shoulder abducted approximately 70°.

C. Extend the opposite arm fully at chest height in a punch-out position. Keep the spine in its neutral position, but allow the torso to turn slightly away from midline on the tubing side.

D. Press out with the resisted arm fully in the low or high plane of motion while bending the opposite arm, driving the elbow back. The torso should turn in the opposite motion as in the starting position. The eyes should focus in front of the foot of the lead leg. The starting lunge stance must be maintained, but the hip of the back leg should naturally rotate inward while the heel lifts slightly. The rib cage should be lifted high, lower spine neutral (not rounded), and bellybutton drawn toward spine.

E. Slowly return to the starting position. Place handle in opposite hand, change foot positions, and repeat an equal amount of repetitions.

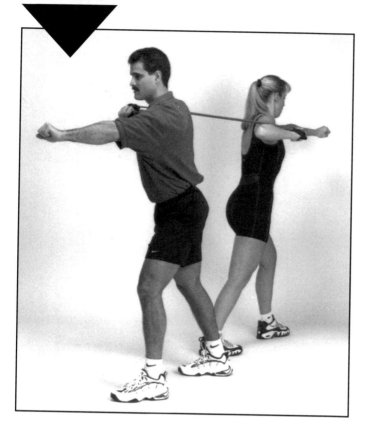

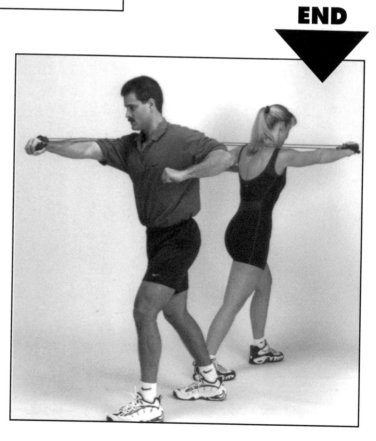

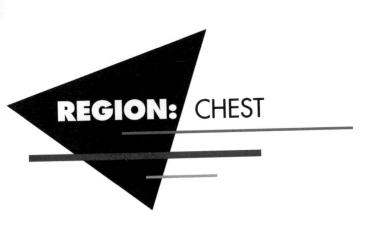

REGION: CHEST

XERTUBE STANDING SINGLE ARM INCLINE CHEST PRESS

(Pectorals)

A. Anchor tubing between ankle and knee height when standing. Face away from attachment site and align tubing slightly outside shoulder of exercising arm.

B. Move away from attachment site to desired tension level and assume a staggered lunge stance with leg opposite the exercising arm forward. Keep knees bent slightly, hips back, pelvis tilted slightly anterior, lumbar spine neutral, and lean torso forward slightly. Grasp handle(s) in hand with thumb up and positioned parallel to lower chest (low position) with shoulder abducted approximately 30°. One may also position the hand with palm down, parallel to lower chest (high position) with shoulder abducted approximately 75°.

C. Extend the opposite arm fully at chest height in a punch-out position. Keep the spine in its neutral position, but allow the torso to turn slightly away from midline on the tubing side.

D. Press out and up with the resisted arm so that the hand finishes just above shoulder height while simultaneously bending the opposite arm, driving the elbow back in a reciprocal motion. The torso should turn in the opposite motion as in the starting position. The eyes should focus in front of the foot of the lead leg. The starting lunge stance must be maintained, but the hip of the back leg should naturally rotate internally while the heel lifts slightly. The rib cage should be lifted high, lumbar curvature neutral (not rounded), and bellybutton drawn toward spine.

E. Slowly return to the starting position. Move the body so that the opposite arm is positioned correctly and repeat an equal amount of repetitions.

START
30°

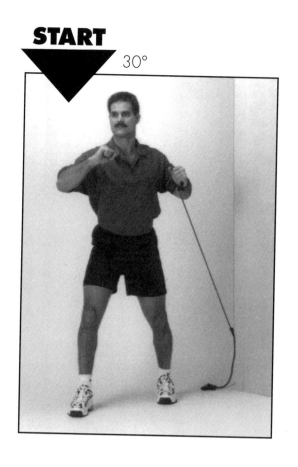

END
30°

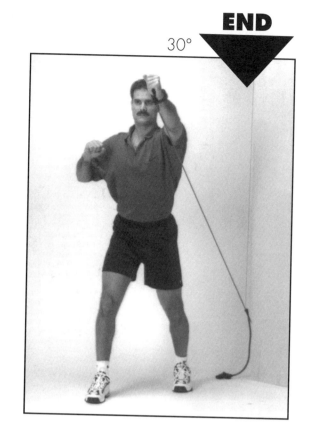

START
70°

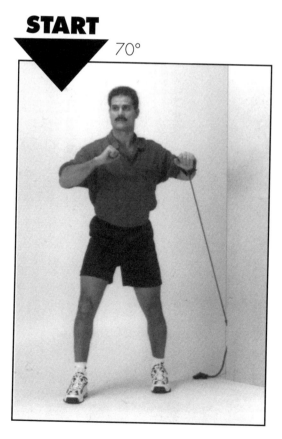

END
70°

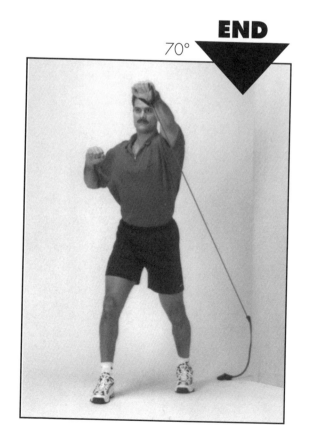

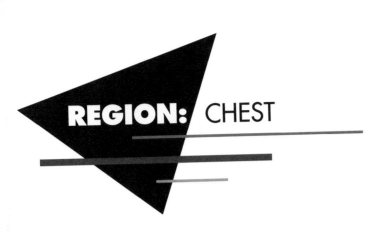

XERTUBE STANDING SINGLE ARM CHEST FLYE

(Pectorals)

A. Anchor tubing at shoulder height, grasp or place palm of one open exercising hand against handle with thumb up. Place opposite hand on opposite hip.

B. Turn so exercising arm is parallel to and just in front of tubing insertion with arm straight out from and slightly behind shoulder.

C. Assume a square stance slightly wider than shoulder width. Assume a 1/4 squat position, keep knees bent slightly, hips back, pelvis tilted slightly anterior, lumbar spine neutral and lean torso forward slightly.

D. Keep wrist firm and arm straight with a slight bend in elbow while pushing into midline of body.

E. 1. Hand ends extended out from mid chest in a thumbs up position.

   2. For an advanced movement pattern, gradually rotate inward from shoulder joint drawing arm across lower chest ending with thumb facing midline.

F. Keep the chest up, rib cage lifted, bellybutton drawn toward spine, and the lumbar spine in its neutral curvature.

G. Turn the opposite direction and repeat equal amount of repetitions with other hand.

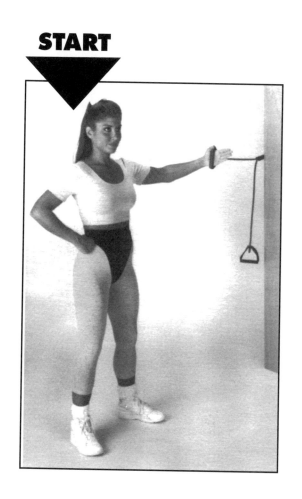

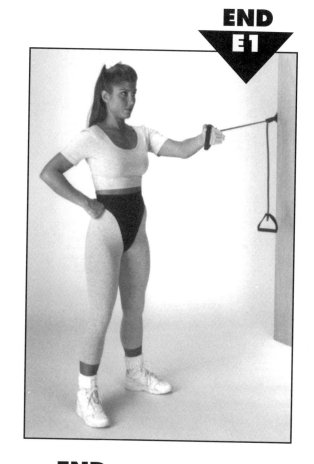

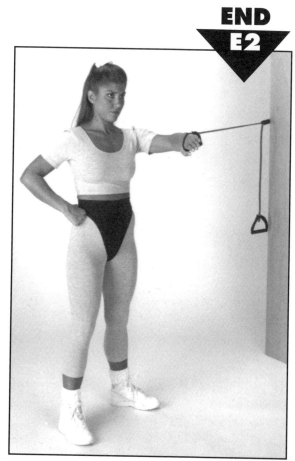

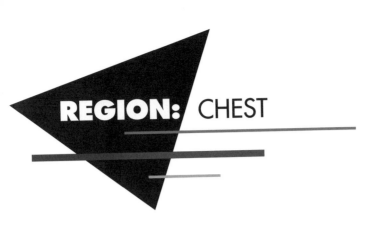

XERTUBE PARTNER STANDING SINGLE ARM CHEST FLYE

(Pectorals)

A. Exerciser and partner stand next to each other and align right shoulders. Each person grasps one handle with the right hand.

B. Move away from each other taking steps laterally to a desired tension level and assume a quarter squat position. Keep hips back, pelvis tilted slightly anterior, lumbar spine neutral, and lean torso forward slightly (athletic position). Position handle(s) in the back portion of the hand using a cupped grip and place opposite hand on hip. Take a small step forward so that the exercising hand is slightly behind shoulder with thumb up and palm facing forward. One should feel a slight stretch in the upper pectoral and anterior shoulder region.

C. Keep the elbow soft and gradually adduct and straighten the arm in a horizontal pattern. Finish with the hand open and at height of lower chest with thumb up. Keep the chest up, rib cage lifted, bellybutton drawn toward spine and the spine in its neutral curvature.

D. Slowly reverse this pattern to the starting position. Turn the opposite direction, align the exercising hand slightly behind shoulder, and repeat an equal amount of repetitions with the opposite arm.

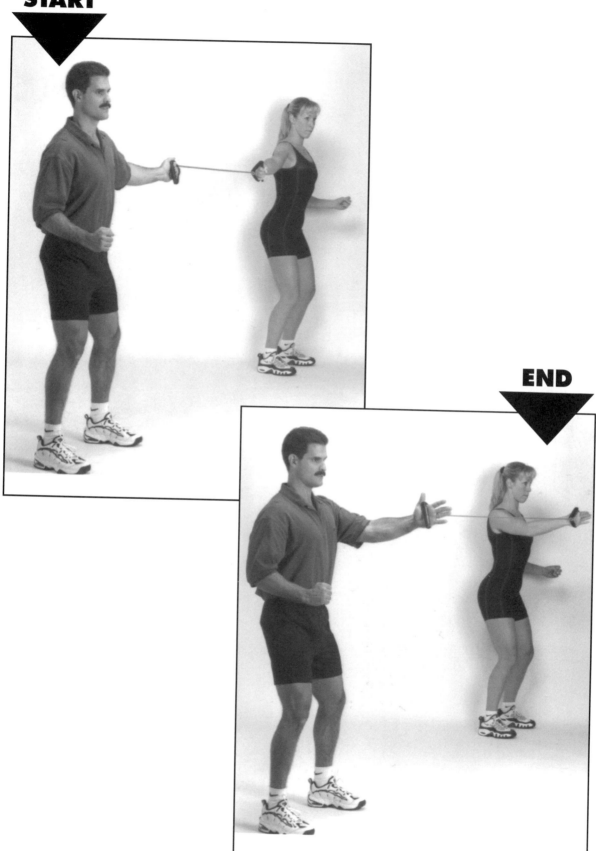

END

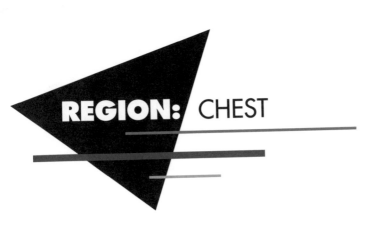

REGION: CHEST

XERTUBE STANDING SINGLE ARM CHEST FLYE (Upward Arc)

(Pectorals)

A. Anchor tubing at ankle height and position torso parallel to and forward of attachment site approximately 12".

B. Grasp handle(s) in hand closest to attachment site. Position the handle(s) in the back portion of the hand using a cupped grip and place opposite hand on hip. Move away from attachment site to desired tension level and assume a quarter squat position. Keep hips back, pelvis tilted slightly anterior, lumbar spine neutral, and torso slightly forward (athletic position). Keep torso square with the arm straightened at approximately 30° abduction and slightly behind the shoulder with palm facing forward. One should feel a slight stretch in the upper pectoral and anterior shoulder region.

C. Keep the elbow soft and wrist firm while gradually adducting and straightening arm in an upward diagonal pattern. Finish with the hand open and at height of lower chest with thumb pointing up and palm facing midline. Keep the chest up, rib cage lifted, bellybutton drawn toward spine, and the spine in its neutral curvature. The quarter squat athletic position must be maintained.

D. Slowly reverse this pattern to the starting position. Turn the opposite direction and repeat an equal amount of repetitions with the opposite arm.

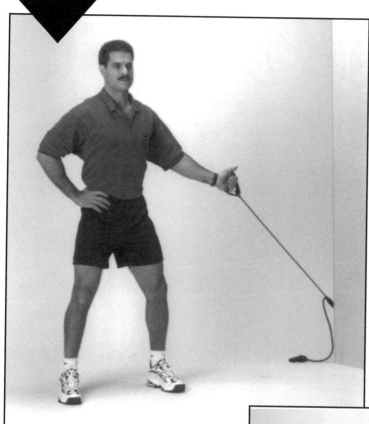

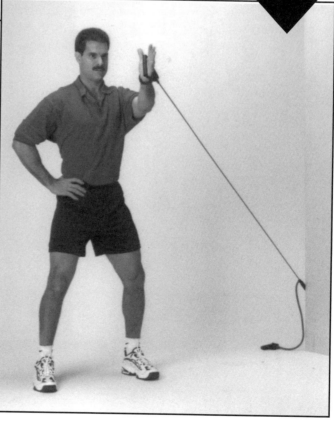

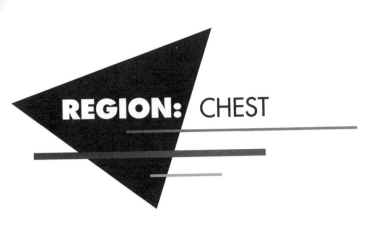

STEP XERTUBE STANDING SINGLE ARM INCLINE CHEST PRESS

(PECTORALS)

A. Tubing is secured through step strap at outside attachment. Stand at end of step furthest away from step strap.

B. Face away from attachment site and align tubing slightly outside shoulder of exercising arm. Assume a staggered lunge stance with foot opposite the exercising arm forward and other foot directly over middle of step block. For safety, use only one block under each end of step. Keep knees bent slightly, hips back, pelvis tilted slightly anterior, lower spine neutral, and lean torso forward slightly. Grasp handle(s) in hand with palm down, parallel to lower chest with shoulder abducted approximately 75°.

C. Extend the opposite arm fully at chest height in a punch-out position. Keep the spine in its neutral position, but allow the torso to turn slightly away from midline on the tubing side.

D. Press out and up with the resisted arm so that the hand finishes just above shoulder height while bending the opposite arm, driving the elbow back in a reciprocal motion. The torso should turn in the opposite motion as in the starting position. The starting lunge stance must be maintained and the eyes should focus forward of the foot of the lead leg. The rib cage should be lifted high, lumbar curvature neutral (not rounded), and bellybutton drawn toward spine.

E. Slowly return to the starting position. Move the body so that the opposite arm is positioned correctly and repeat an equal amount of repetitions.

> ### TECH TIPS
> **If end of step attachment site rises during the pushing motion, move foot on step toward attachment site.**

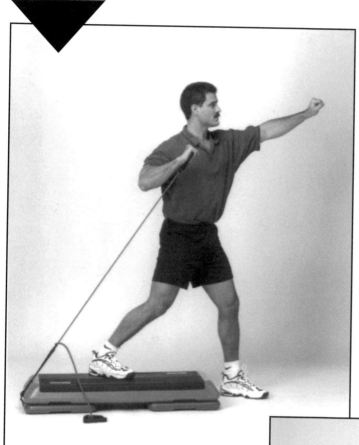

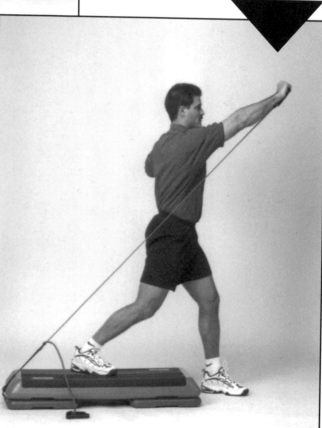

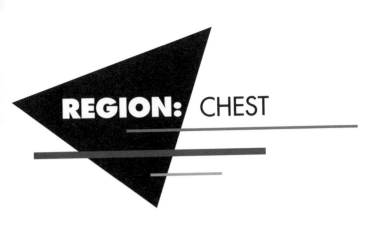

REGION: CHEST

STEP XERTUBE STANDING SINGLE ARM CHEST FLYE (Upward Arc)

(Pectorals)

A. Tubing is secured through step strap at outside attachment. Stand at end of step farthest from step strap.

B. Position torso parallel to and forward of attachment site approximately 12". Place the foot nearest to step directly over middle of step block and place other foot on floor. For safety, use only one block under each end of step

C. Grasp handle(s) in hand closest to attachment site. Position the handle(s) in the back portion of the hand using a cupped grip. Place opposite hand on hip and assume a quarter squat position. Keep hips back, pelvis tilted slightly anterior, lumbar spine neutral, and torso slightly forward (athletic position). Keep torso square with the arm straightened at approximately 30° abduction and slightly behind the shoulder with palm facing forward. One should feel a slight stretch in the upper pectoral and anterior shoulder region.

D. Keep the elbow soft and wrist firm while gradually adducting and straightening arm in an upward diagonal pattern. Finish with the hand open and at height of lower chest with thumb pointing up and palm facing midline. Keep the chest up, rib cage lifted, bellybutton drawn toward spine, and the spine in its neutral curvature. The quarter squat athletic position must be maintained.

E. Slowly reverse this pattern to the starting position. Turn the opposite direction and repeat an equal amount of repetitions with the opposite arm.

> ### TECH TIPS
> **If end of step attachment site rises during the pushing motion, move foot on step toward attachment site.**

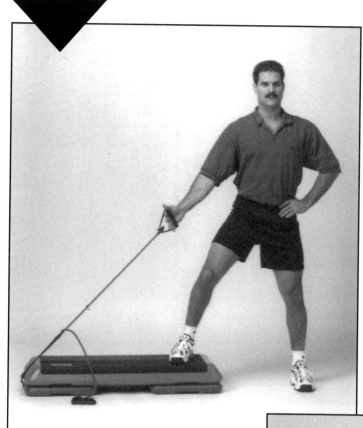

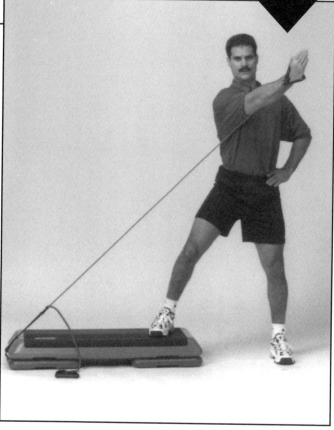

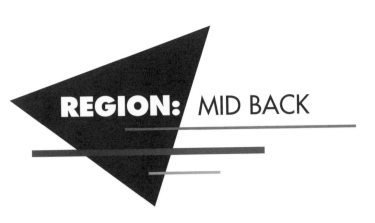

XERTUBE SEATED ROW (HIGH ROW AND LOW ROW)

(Middle Trapezius/Rhomboids/Latissimus Dorsi)

A. Sit with knees comfortably bent, center tubing under middle of both feet. Grasp tubing in between both feet and pull toward you to create a loop. Place loop back over feet.

B. Keep feet together for less resistance and apart for more resistance.

C. Grasp handles with palms down (high row) or palms up (low row). Sit up with a slight lean forward, keeping a natural arch in lower back. Arms should be fully extended.

D. HIGH ROW - With firm wrists, bend elbows, pull hands up and back while gradually flaring elbows. Elbows finish at shoulder height.

LOW ROW - With firm wrists, bend elbows and pull back so little fingers contact lower rib cage. Elbows finish behind torso.

E. Finish with chest expanded, rib cage lifted, lumbar spine neutral and bellybutton drawn toward spine. Upper and lower arms should form 90° angles and shoulder blades should be squeezed back and together.

TECH TIPS

The Latissimus Dorsi is utilized to a higher degree when performing the low row (increased shoulder extension).

The Rhomboids and Middle Trapezius are utilized to a higher degree when performing the high row (shoulder horizontal adduction).

This exercise may also be performed by anchoring tubing at ankle height. Sit with knees comfortably bent and perform steps C through E.

This exercise may also be performed by anchoring tubing at chest height.

Stand in a staggered lunge position or square stance and perform steps C through E.

START

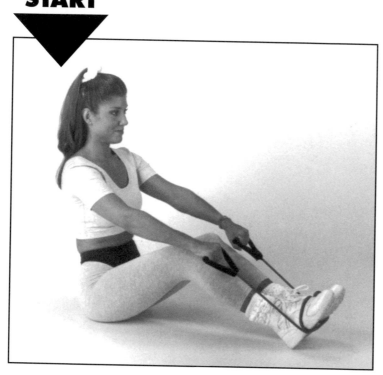

END HIGH ROW

END LOW ROW

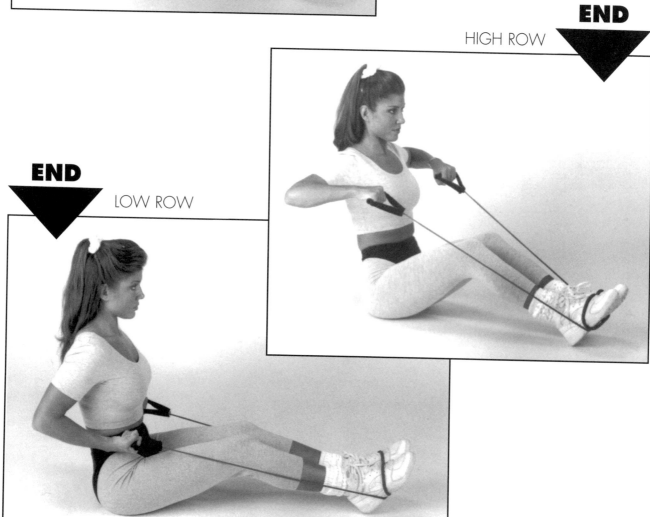

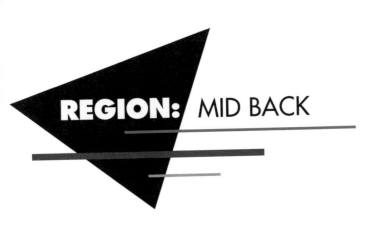

XERTUBE STANDING HIGH ROW
(Rhomboids, Middle Trapezius)

A. Anchor tubing at lower chest height while standing with torso facing attachment site.

B. Grasp handle in each hand and move away from attachment site to desired tension level and assume a quarter squat position. Keep hips back, pelvis tilted slightly anterior, lumbar spine neutral, and lean torso forward slightly (athletic position). Extend arm fully with palm facing down.

C. With firm wrists, pull back and slightly out while expanding the chest and lifting the rib cage. Finish with eyes focused forward, wrists just outside lower chest, arms at 90° angles, shoulders abducted approximately 70°, shoulder blades squeezed together, and bellybutton drawn toward spine. The quarter-squat athletic position must be maintained throughout.

D. Slowly return to the starting position.

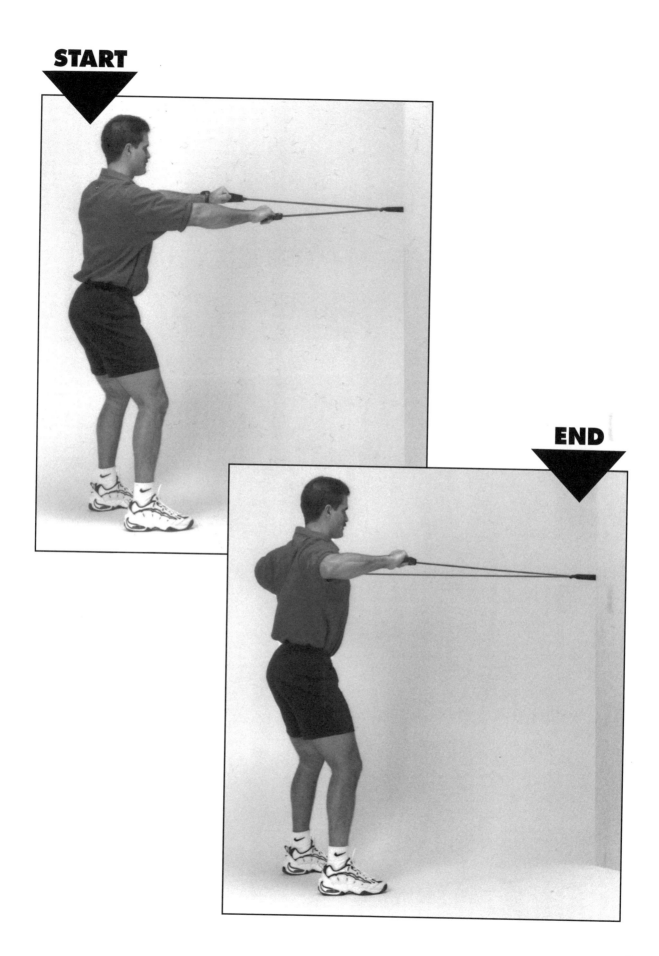

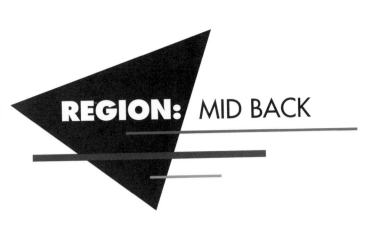
XERTUBE PARTNER STANDING HIGH ROW
(Rhomboids, Middle Trapezius)

A. Exerciser stands facing partner. Two Xertubes are used simultaneously for this exercise. Each person grasps one handle of the same Xertube with the right hand and one handle of the other Xertube with the left.

B. Move away from each other taking steps backward to desired tension level and assume a quarter-squat position. Keep hips back, pelvis tilted slightly anterior, spine neutral, and lean torso forward slightly (athletic position). Extend arms fully just below shoulder height with palms facing down.

C. With firm wrists, pull back and slightly out while expanding the chest and lifting the rib cage. Finish with eyes focused forward, wrists just outside lower chest, arms at 90° angles, shoulders abducted approximately 70°, shoulder blades squeezed together, and bellybutton drawn toward spine. The quarter-squat athletic position must be maintained throughout.

D. Slowly return to the starting position.

**This exercise may be performed with one arm only or in an alternating arm fashion.

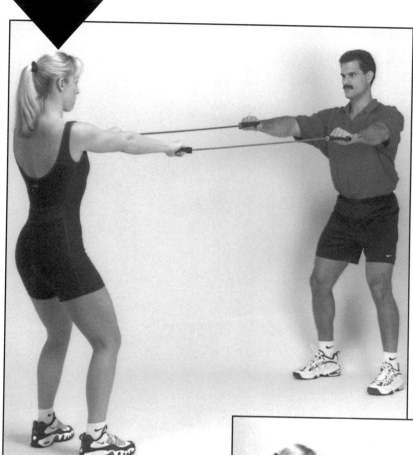

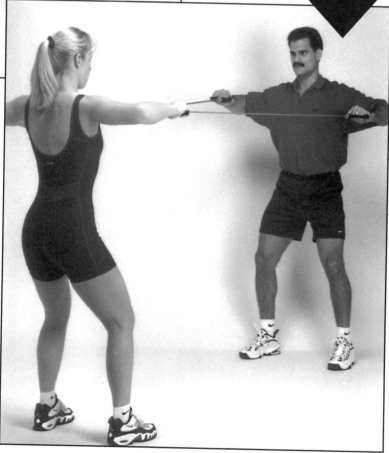

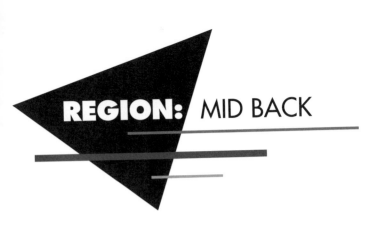

XERTUBE STANDING SINGLE ARM HIGH ROW

(Rhomboids, Middle Trapezius)

A. Anchor tubing at lower chest height when standing. Face tubing with shoulder of exercising arm aligned slightly inside attachment site.

B. Grasp handle(s) in hand and move away from attachment site to desired tension level and assume a quarter-squat position. Keep hips back, pelvis tilted slightly anterior, spine neutral, and lean torso forward slightly (athletic position). Extend arm fully with palm facing down and position other arm next to upper rib cage with arm bent 90°. Keep the spine in its neutral position, but allow the torso to rotate slightly toward midline on the pulling side.

C. With a firm wrist, pull back and slightly out while expanding the chest and lifting the rib cage. Simultaneously extend the other arm fully in a punching action. Finish with eyes focused forward, wrist just outside lower chest, arm at 90° angle, shoulder abducted approximately 70°, shoulder blade squeezed toward spine, and bellybutton drawn toward spine. The torso should rotate one-quarter turn away from midline on the pulling side. The quarter-squat athletic position must be maintained.

D. Slowly return to the starting position. Position the other shoulder slightly inside attachment site and repeat an equal amount of repetitions.

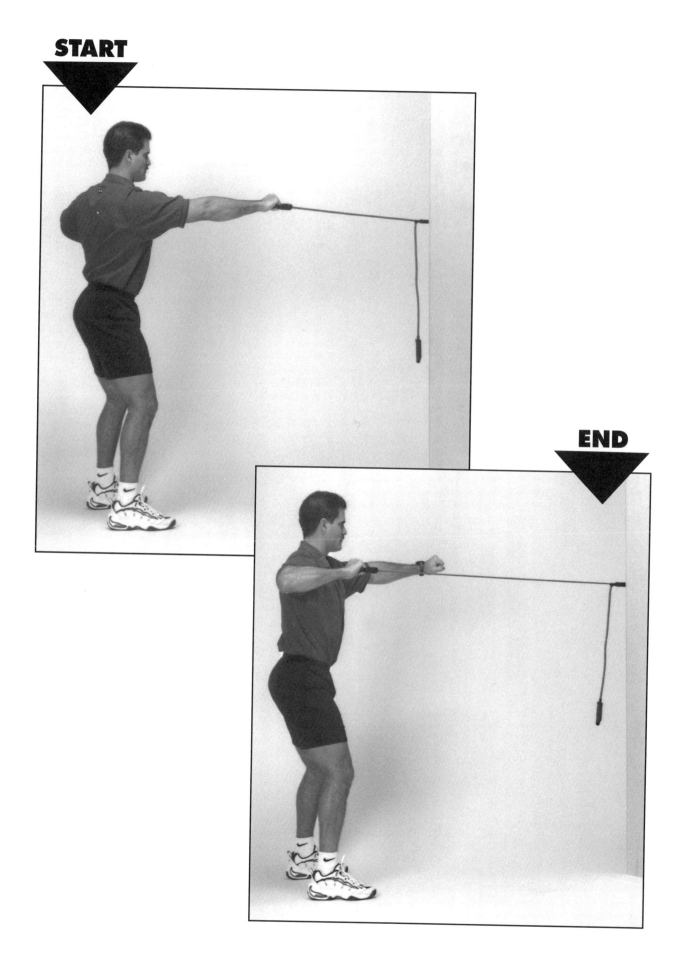

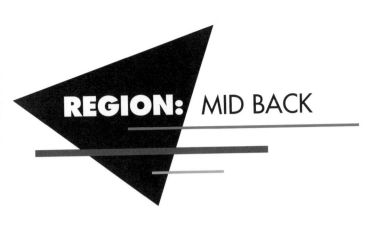

XERTUBE STANDING LOW ROW

(Latissimus Dorsi)

A. Anchor tubing just above waist height while standing with torso facing attachment site.

B. Grasp a handle in each hand and move away from attachment site to desired tension level and assume a quarter-squat position. Keep hips back, pelvis tilted slightly anterior, lumbar spine neutral, and lean torso forward slightly (athletic position). Extend arms fully with palms facing each other.

C. With firm wrists, pull back while expanding the chest and lifting the rib cage. Finish with eyes focused forward, wrists just outside lower rib cage, arms at 90° angles, shoulder blades squeezed together, and bellybutton drawn toward spine. The quarter-squat athletic position must be maintained throughout.

D. Slowly return to the starting position.

START

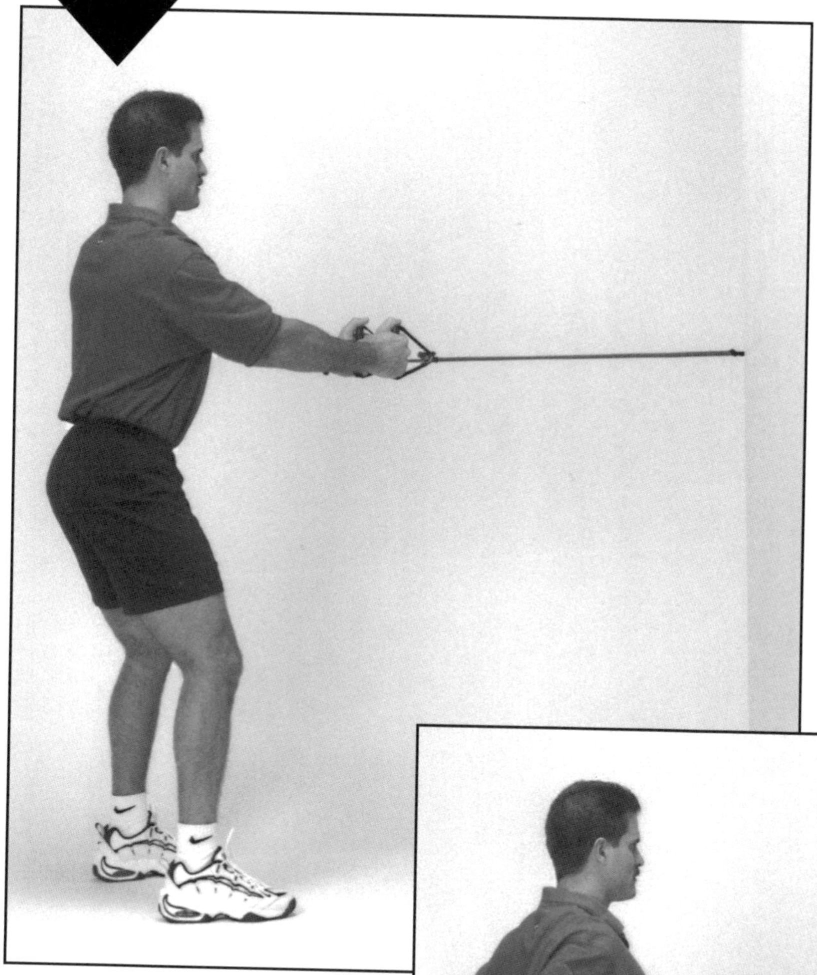

END

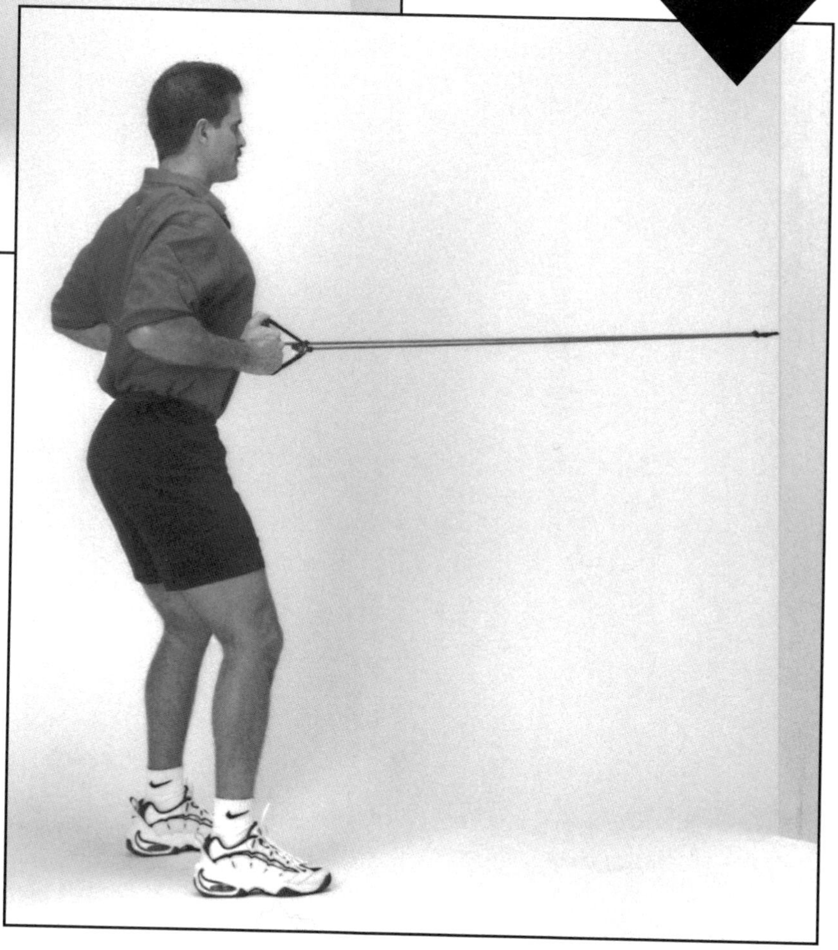

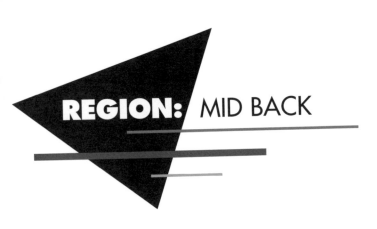

XERTUBE PARTNER STANDING LOW ROW

(Latissimus Dorsi)

A. Exerciser stands facing partner. Two Xertubes are used simultaneously for this exercise. Each person grasps one handle of the same Xertube with the right hand and one handle of the other Xertube with the left hand.

B. Move away from each other taking steps backward to a desired tension level and assume a quarter-squat position. Keep hips back, pelvis tilted slightly anterior, lumbar spine neutral, and lean torso forward slightly (athletic position). Extend arms fully with hands parallel to lower rib cage and palms facing each other.

C. With firm wrists, pull back while expanding the chest and lifting the rib cage. Finish with eyes focused forward, wrists just outside lower rib cage, arms at 90° angles, shoulder blades squeezed together, and bellybutton drawn toward spine. The quarter-squat athletic position must be maintained throughout.

D. Slowly return to the starting position.

**This exercise may be performed with one arm only or in an alternative arm fashion.

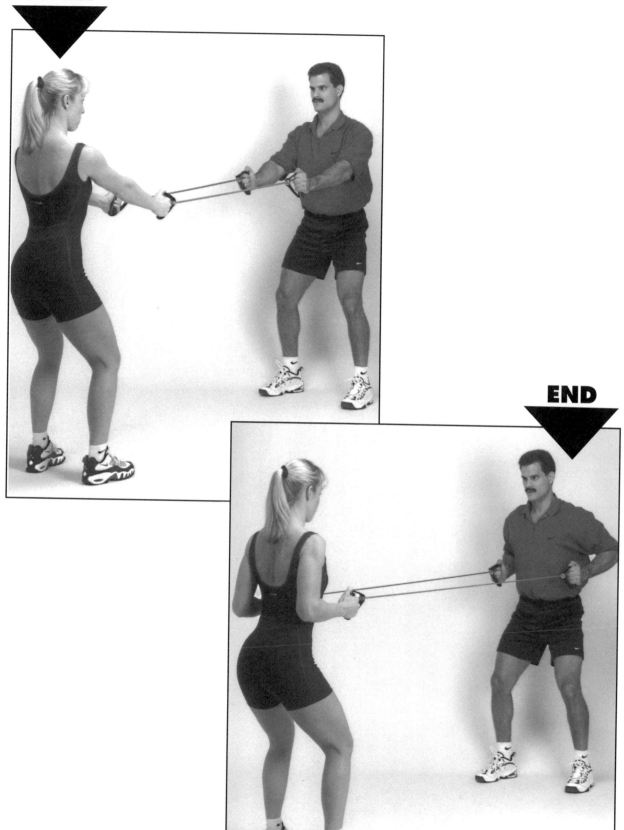

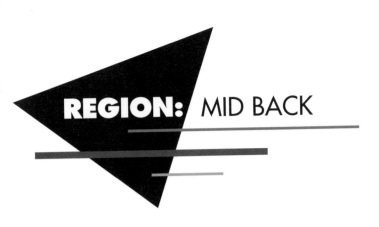
XERTUBE STANDING SINGLE ARM LOW ROW

(Latissimus Dorsi)

A. Anchor tubing just above waist height while standing. Face tubing with shoulder of exercising arm aligned with attachment site.

B. Grasp handle(s) in hand and move away from attachment site to desired tension level and assume a quarter-squat position. Keep hips back, pelvis tilted slightly anterior, lumbar spine neutral, and lean torso forward slightly (athletic position). Extend arm fully with palm facing midline and position other arm next to lower rib cage with arm bent 90°. Allow the torso to rotate slightly toward midline on the pulling side.

C. With a firm wrist, pull back while expanding the chest and lifting the rib cage. Simultaneously extend the other arm fully in a punching action. Finish with the wrist just outside the lower rib cage, arm at 90° angle, shoulder blade squeezed toward spine, and bellybutton drawn toward spine. The torso should rotate one-quarter away from the midline on the pulling side. The quarter-squat athletic position must be maintained.

D. Slowly return to the starting position. Position the other shoulder slightly inside attachment site and repeat an equal amount of repetitions.

START

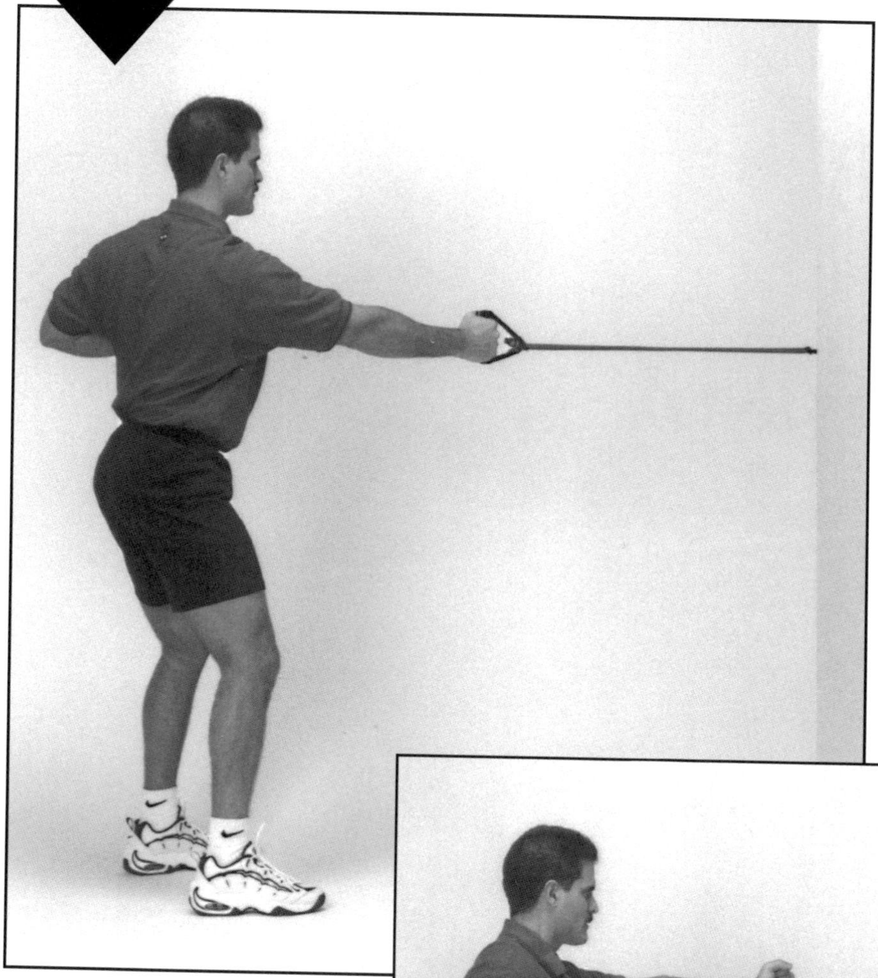

END

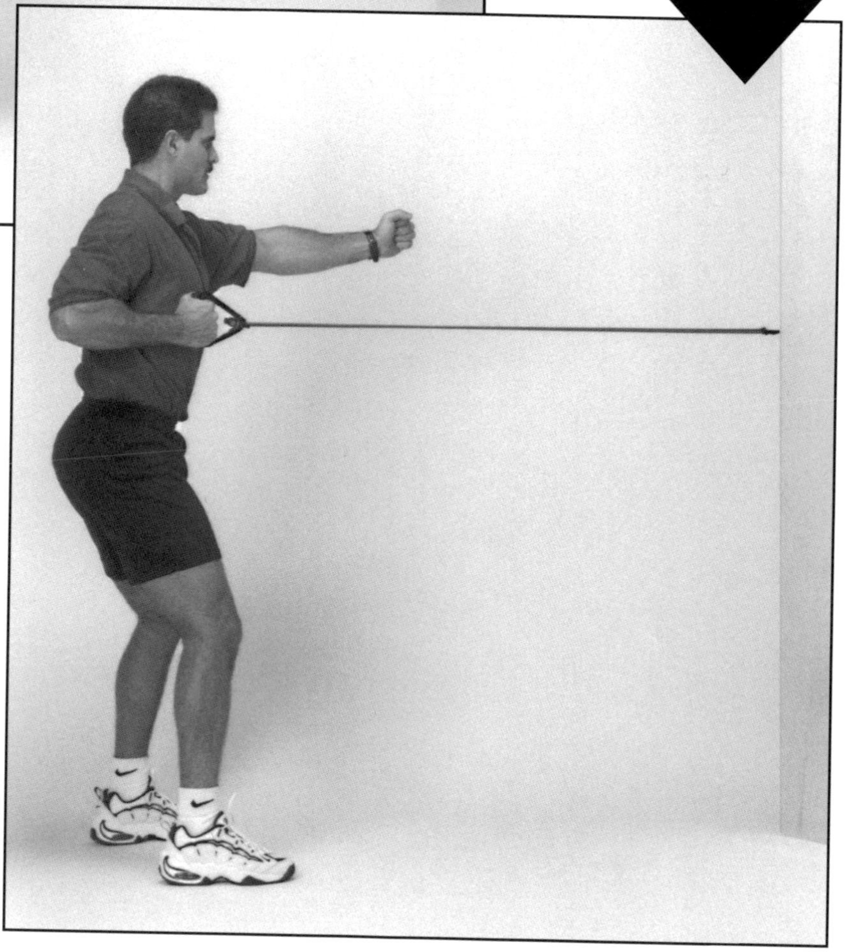

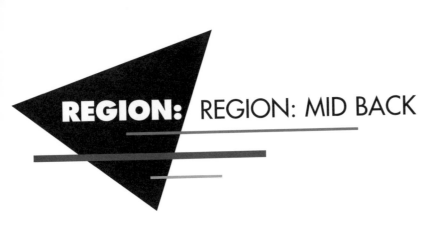

XERTUBE BENT OVER SINGLE ARM LOW ROW

(Latissimus Dorsi)

A. Anchor tubing at ankle height. Face tubing with shoulder of exercising arm aligned with attachment site.

B. Grasp handle(s) in hand and move away from attachment site to desired tension level and assume a staggered lunge stance with leg opposite the exercising arm forward. Place uninvolved hand on knee, bend knees, and lower torso to approximately 45° in relation to floor. Extend exercising arm fully while keeping the lumbar spine in its neutral position (not rounded).

C. With a firm wrist, pull back while expanding the chest and lifting the rib cage. Allow the torso to turn slightly away from midline on the tubing side. Finish with the wrist just outside the lower rib cage, arm at 90° angle, shoulder blade squeezed toward spine, and bellybutton drawn toward spine. The eyes should focus forward of the lead leg. The starting lunge stance and torso position must be maintained.

D. Slowly return to the starting position. Position the other arm in line with the attachment site and repeat an equal amount of repetitions.

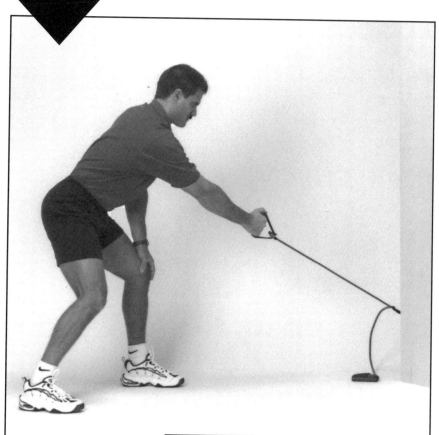

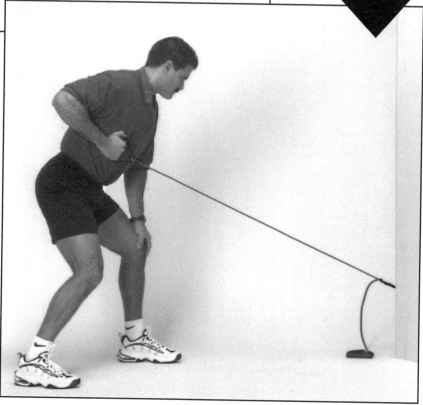

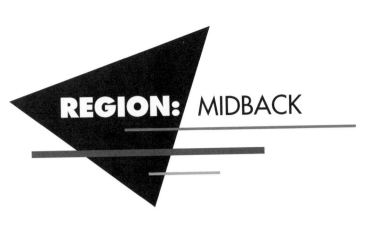

STEP XERTUBE BENT OVER SINGLE ARM LOW ROW

(Latissimus Dorsi)

A. Tubing is secured through step strap at outside attachment.

B. Grasp one handle and stand on step farthest from step strap.

C. Take a drop step to the floor with the same side foot as the hand holding the handle. This position should reflect a narrow staggered lunge stance. Soften the knees, tilt pelvis slightly anterior, keep hips back and lumbar spine neutral.

D. The shoulder of the exercising arm should be aligned with attachment site.

E. Place uninvolved hand on one knee, lower torso to approximately 45° in relation to the floor. Extend exercising arm fully while keeping the lumbar spine in its neutral position (not rounded).

F. With a firm wrist, pull back while expanding the chest and lifting the rib cage. Allow the torso to turn slightly away from mid-line on the tubing side. Finish with the wrist just outside the lower rib cage at a 90° angle, shoulder blade squeezed toward spine and bellybutton drawn toward spine. The eyes should focus forward of the lead leg. The starting lunge stance and torso position must be maintained.

G. Slowly return to the starting position. Switch foot positions and align the other arm with the attachment site and repeat an equal amount of repetitions.

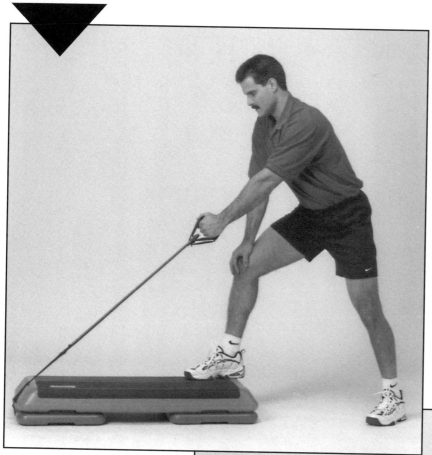

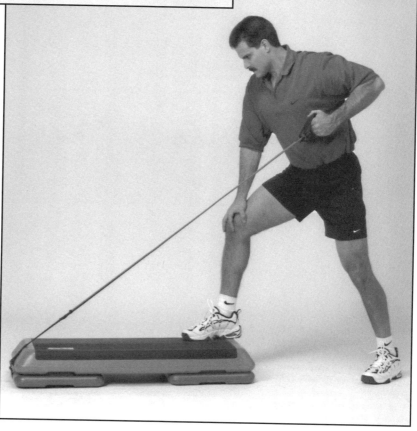

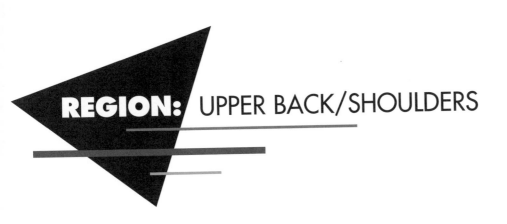
XERTUBE STANDING OVERHEAD PRESS
(Upper Trapezius/Anterior Deltoid/Medial Deltoid)

A. Stand in a narrow staggered lunge position. Place tubing under arch of rear foot and soften both knees. Keep hips back, pelvis tilted slightly anterior and lumbar spine neutral.

B. Grasp handles and bring hands up to a comfortable position just in front of shoulders.

C. Abduct upper arms about 30° away from torso with thumbs pointing at front portion of shoulders.

D. Press upward and back, keeping wrists firm, and finish with hands directly over shoulders.

E. Keep the chest up, rib cage lifted, bellybutton drawn toward spine and the lumbar spine in its neutral curvature.

> **TECH TIPS**
>
> **This exercise may be performed one arm at a time. If the exerciser is unable to stabilize the spine and pelvis, one arm should be used.**

START

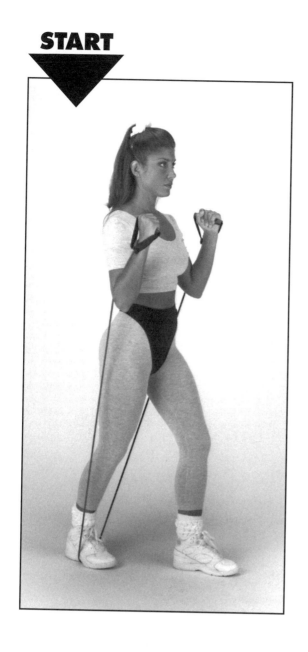

END

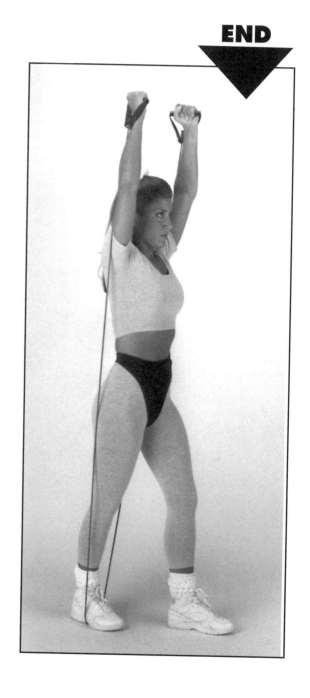

XERTUBE STANDING HALF-SQUAT TO SINGLE ARM OVERHEAD PRESS

(Anterior Deltoid, Medial Deltoid)

A. Place tubing horizontal on floor. Step on middle of tubing with ball of one foot.

B. Grasp handle with hand on same side as foot stepping on tubing. Bend elbow and bring hand just in front of shoulder. The thumb should point at the front portion of the shoulder with the upper arm abducted approximately 30°.

**Move tubing toward the exercising arm side to decrease tension or toward the uninvolved side to increase tension.

C. Place feet approximately shoulder width apart. Lead with hips and perform a half-squat. Keep wrist firm, press upward and slightly back while simultaneously rising from the half-squat and finish with the hand directly over shoulder with palm facing midline. The rib cage should be lifted, bellybutton drawn toward spine and the lumbar spine in its neutral curvature.

D. Slowly return to the starting position. Place the tubing under the other foot and repeat an equal amount of repetitions.

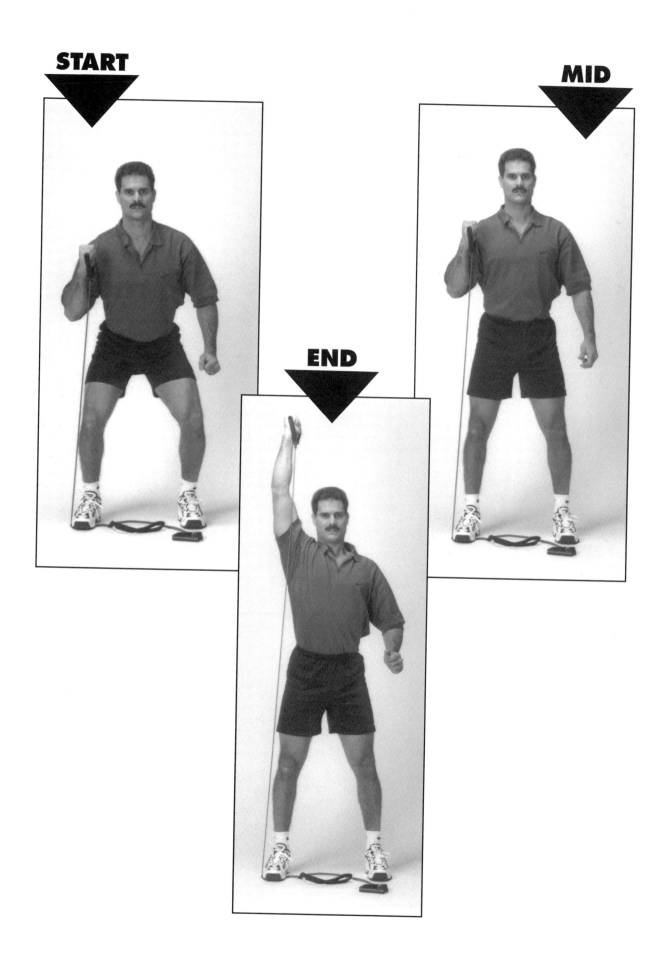

START

MID

END

XERTUBE STANDING UPRIGHT ROW
(Upper Trapezius/Medial Deltoid)

A. Stand in a staggered, narrow or wide stance. Place tubing under arch of front foot or both feet and soften knees. Keep hips back, pelvis tilted slightly anterior and lumbar spine neutral.

B. Grasp handles with palms of hands facing thighs, allowing arms to hang straight down from shoulders. To increase upper trapezius recruitment, perform a modified half-shrug (scapular elevation).

C. Bend and flare elbows and immediately face palms toward floor. Hands are kept at elbow height as they are moved away from sides of body. Upper and lower arms move as one unit and wrists remain firm.

D. Elbows should be at same height as hands and parallel to shoulders. End with upper and lower arms forming 90° angles.

E. Keep the chest up, rib cage lifted, bellybutton drawn toward spine, and the lumbar spine in its neutral curvature.

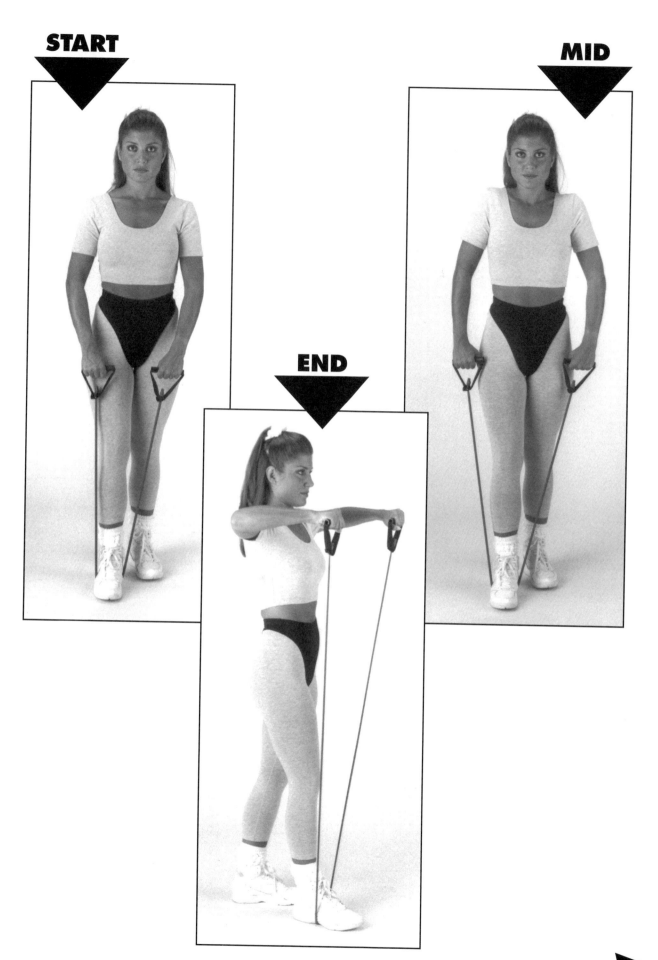

START

MID

END

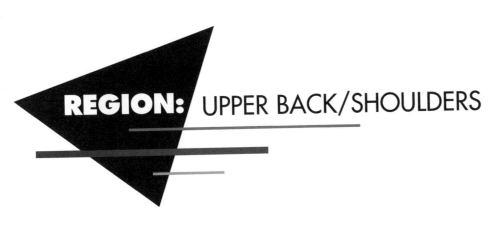

XERTUBE STANDING SHRUG
(Upper Trapezius)

A. Stand in a staggered, narrow or wide stance. Place tubing under each arch of front foot or both feet and soften knees. Keep hips back, pelvis tilted slightly anterior and lumbar spine neutral.

B. Grasp handles and allow arms to hang down straight from shoulders with palms facing back.

C. Abduct arms approximately 30° from body while shrugging shoulders straight up toward ears.

D. Keep the chest up, rib cage lifted, bellybutton drawn toward spine, and the lumbar spine in its neutral curvature.

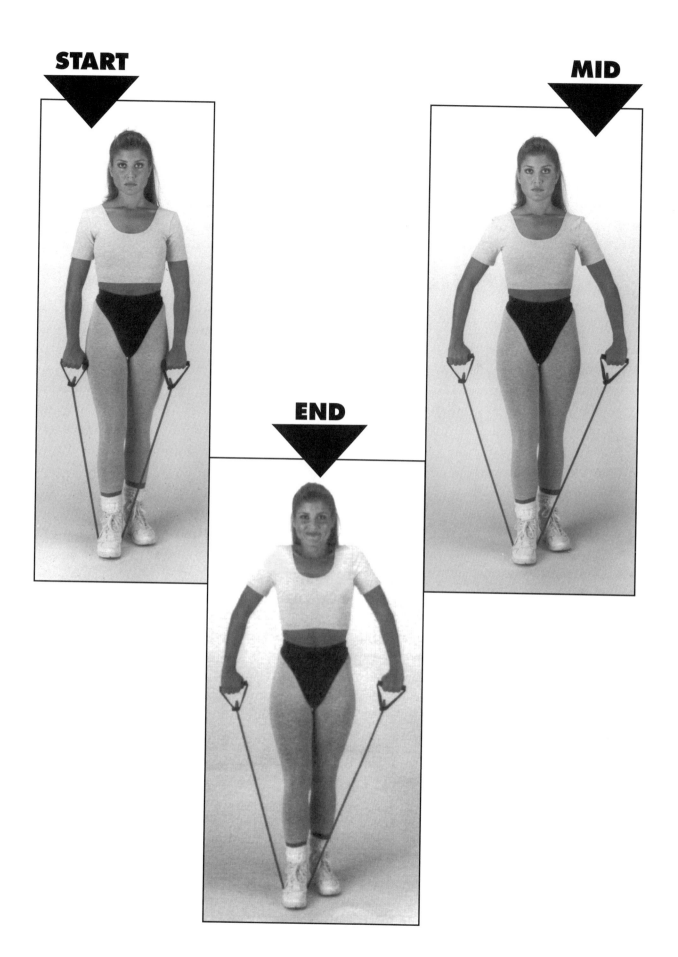

START

MID

END

STEP XERTUBE STANDING OVERHEAD PRESS
(Upper Trapezius/Anterior Deltoid/Medial Deltoid)

A. Tubing is secured through step strap at outside attachment.

B. Grasp handles and stand in a narrow, staggered lunge position at end of step nearest to step strap.

C. Face away from attachment so that tubing pulls from behind body.

D. Bring hands up to a comfortable position just in front of shoulders.

E. Abduct upper arms approximately 30° away from torso with thumbs pointing at front portion of shoulders. Keep hips back, pelvis tilted slightly anterior and lumbar spine neutral.

F. Press upward and back, keeping wrists firm and finish with hands directly over shoulders.

G. Keep the chest up, rib cage lifted, bellybutton drawn toward spine, and the lumbar spine in its neutral curvature.

TECH TIPS
This exercise may be performed one arm at a time. If the exerciser is unable to stabilize the spine and pelvis, one arm should be used.

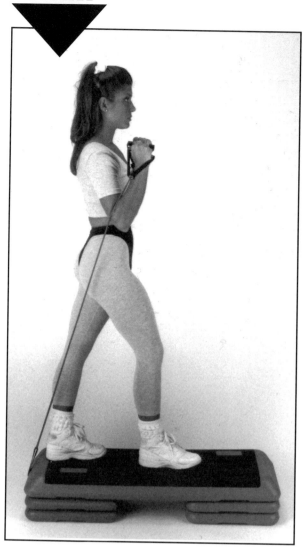

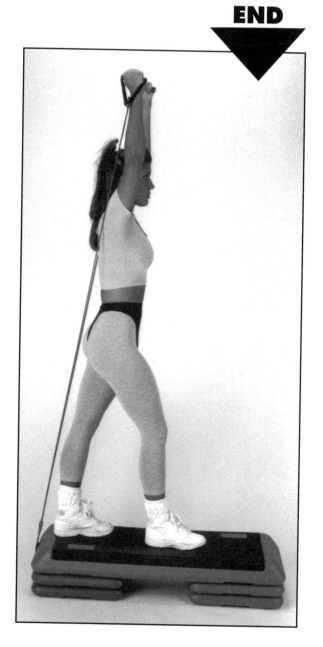

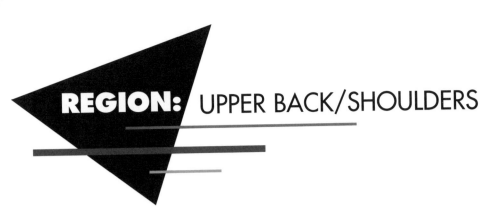

STEP XERTUBE STANDING UPRIGHT ROW
(Upper Trapezius/Medial Deltoid)

A. Tubing is secured through step strap at outside attachment.

B. Grasp handles and stand at end of step nearest to step strap.

C. Face attachment in a narrow, staggered lunge stance and soften knees. Keep hips back, pelvis tilted slightly anterior and lumbar spine neutral.

D. Start with palms of hands facing thighs, allowing arms to hang straight down from shoulders. To increase upper trapezius recruitment, perform a modified half-shrug (scapular elevation).

E. Bend and flare elbows and immediately face palms toward floor. Hands are kept at elbow height as they are moved away from sides of body. Upper and lower arms move as one unit and wrists remain firm.

F. Elbows should be at same height as hands and parallel to shoulders. End with upper and lower arms forming 90° angles.

G. Keep the chest up, rib cage lifted, bellybutton drawn toward spine, and the lumbar spine in its neutral curvature.

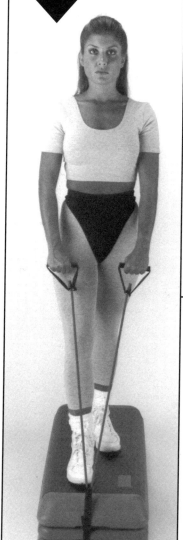

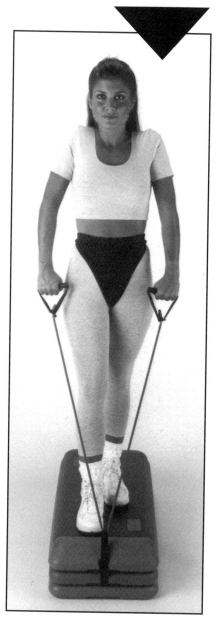

END

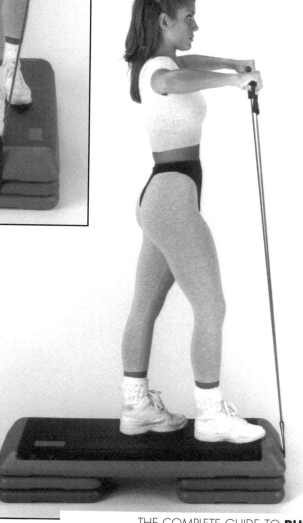

STEP XERTUBE STANDING SHRUG
(Upper Trapezius)

A. Tubing is secured through step strap at outside attachment.

B. Grasp handles and stand in a staggered lunge position at end of step nearest to step strap. Soften knees, keep hips back, tilt pelvis slightly anterior and lumbar spine neutral.

C. Face away from tubing so that tubing pulls from behind body.

D. Allow arms to hang straight down from shoulders with palms facing back.

E. Abduct arms about 30° from body while shrugging shoulders straight upward toward ears.

F. Keep the chest up, rib cage lifted, bellybutton drawn toward spine, and the lumbar spine in its neutral curvature.

END

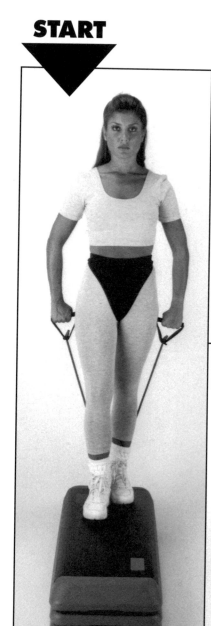

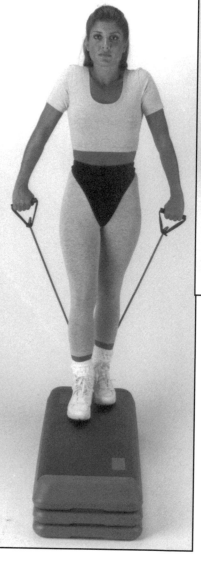

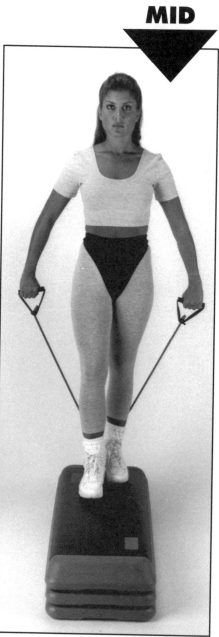

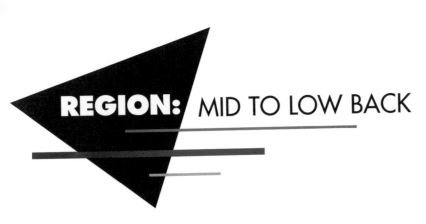

XERTUBE STANDING STRAIGHT ARM PULL DOWN

(Latissimus Dorsi/Lower Trapezius)

A. Anchor tubing just above head height. Place palms of open hands against handles in an overhead position (cupped grip). Back away from insertion until arms fully lengthen.

B. Assume a square stance slightly wider than shoulder width. Extend hips back, soften knees, and draw bellybutton toward spine.

C. Start with hands just above shoulder height. From a straight arm and stiff wrist position, press downward and back until shoulders complete extension. Hands will finish under to slightly behind shoulders.

D. End with chest expanded, rib cage lifted, lumbar spine neutral, and shoulder blades squeezed back and together.

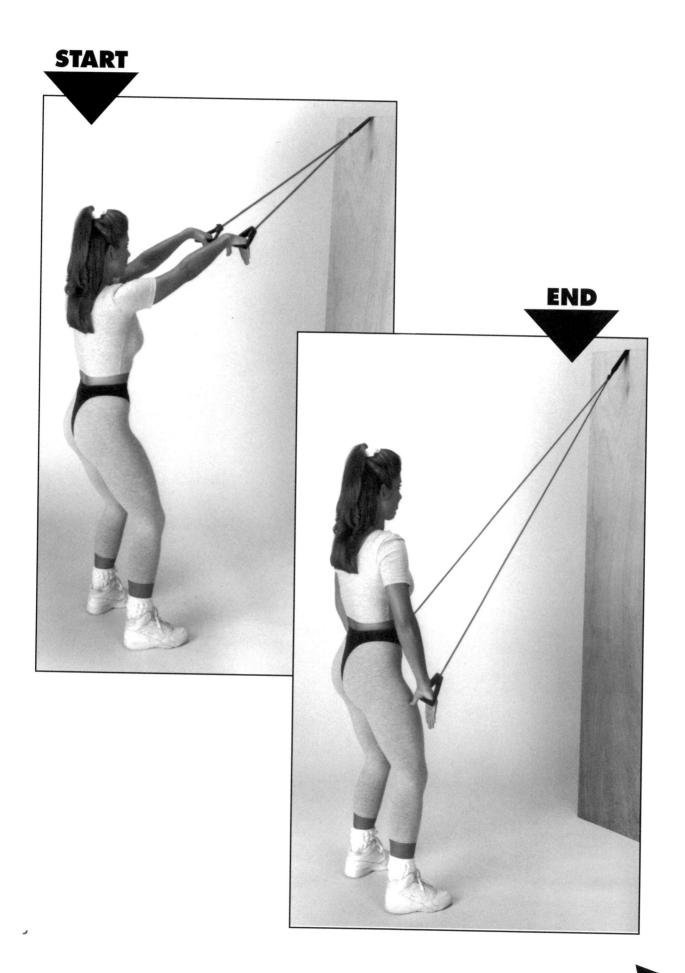

START

END

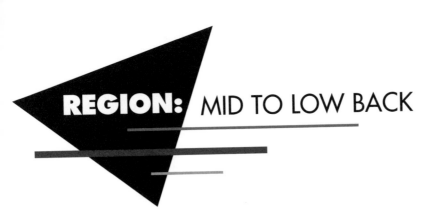

XERTUBE STANDING SINGLE ARM FRONT PULL DOWN

(Latissimus Dorsi/Lower Trapezius)

A. Anchor tubing at top of door when standing. Face tubing with shoulder of exercising arm aligned with attachment site.

B. Grasp handle(s) in hand and move away from attachment site to desired tension level. Assume a staggered lunge stance with the leg opposite the exercising arm forward. Bend knees slightly, keep hips back, tilt pelvis slightly anterior, keep lumbar spine neutral, and lean torso forward slightly. Extend arm fully at approximately 150° of shoulder flexion with palm facing midline. Position other arm next to upper rib cage with arm bent 90°. Allow the torso to rotate slightly toward midline on the pulling side.

C. With a firm wrist, pull down and back while expanding the chest and lifting the rib cage. Simultaneously extend the other arm fully in a punching action. Finish with the wrist just outside the lower chest, arm at 90°, shoulder abducted approximately 30°, shoulder blade squeezed toward spine, and bellybutton drawn toward spine. The torso should rotate one-quarter turn away from midline on the pulling side. The staggered lunge stance must be maintained throughout.

D. Slowly return to the starting position. Position the other arm in line with the attachment site and repeat an equal amount of repetitions.

START

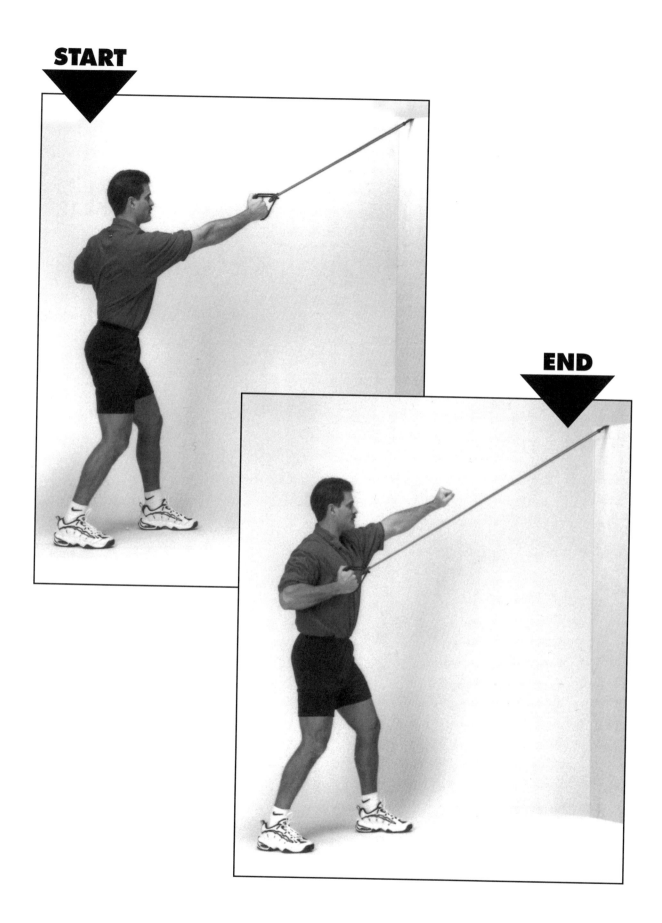

END

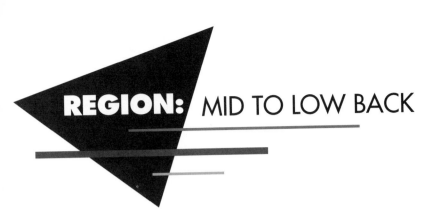

XERTUBE KNEELING BENT ARM PULL DOWN

(Latissimus Dorsi/Lower Trapezius)

A. Anchor tubing just above head height.

B. Grasp handles, back away from insertion until arms are fully lengthened and kneel in a staggered lunge position.

C. Start with hands above shoulder height in a thumbs up position. Lead with elbows driving them down toward waistline, finishing with elbows flared and thumbs contacting hip bones.

D. End with chest expanded, rib cage lifted, lumbar spine neutral, and bellybutton drawn toward spine. The wrists should be kept firm and the shoulder blades should be squeezed back and together.

START

END

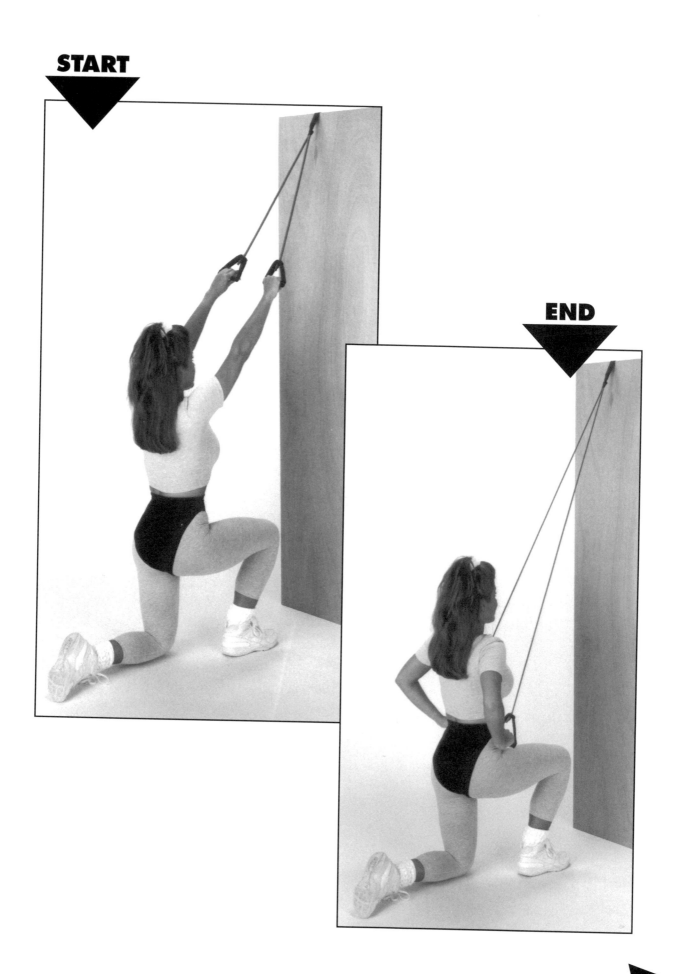

XERTUBE STANDING SINGLE ARM ADDUCTION

(Latissimus Dorsi/Pectorals/Lower Trapezius)

A. Anchor tubing at top of door when standing. Position torso parallel to attachment site.

B. Grasp handle(s) in hand closest to attachment site. Move away from attachment site to desired tension level and assume a quarter-squatquarter-squatand torso slightly forward (athletic position). Position the handle(s) in the back portion of the hand using a cupped grip and place opposite hand on hip. Start with the exercising shoulder just above shoulder height with palm down. Do not allow the shoulder to elevate or shrug.

C. Maintaining a stiff arm position, press downward keeping wrist firm and hand open while expanding the chest and lifting the rib cage. Finish with the hand aligned under the shoulder, palm facing mid-thigh, shoulder blade squeezed toward spine and bellybutton drawn toward spine. The quarter-squat athletic position must be maintained.

D. Slowly return to the starting position. Turn the opposite direction and repeat an equal amount of repetitions.

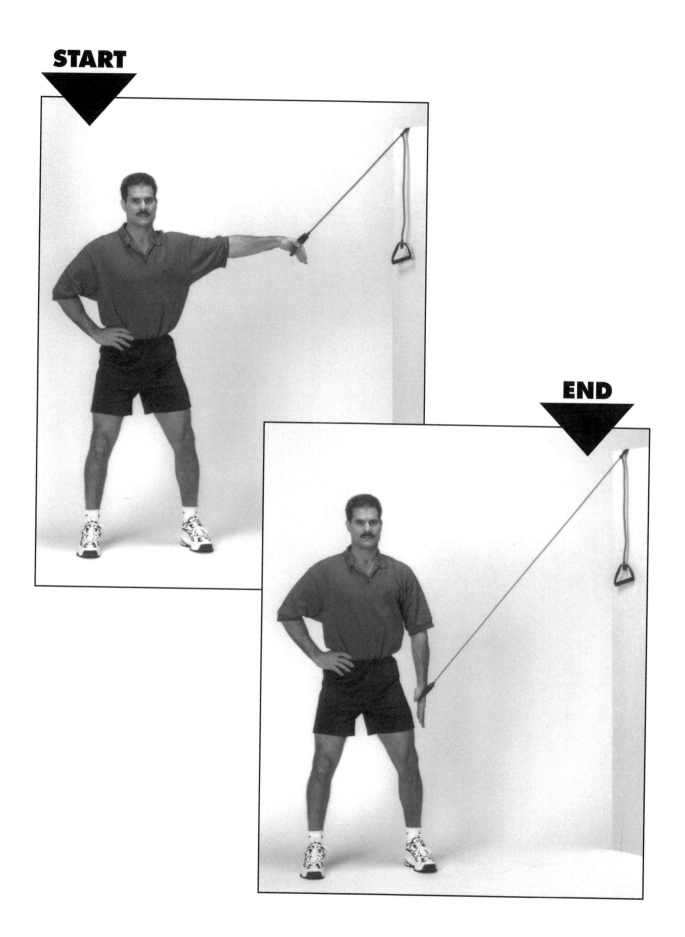

START

END

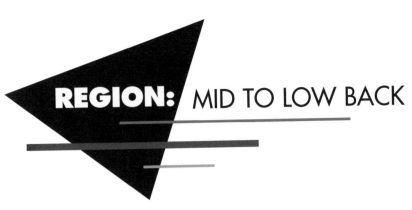

REGION: MID TO LOW BACK

XERTUBE 20°-30° BENCH SUPINE STIFF ARM PULL OVER (LOW ANCHOR)

(Latissimus Dorsi/Lower Trapezius)

A. Anchor tubing at ankle height directly in line with middle of bench. Adjust end of bench closest to attachment site to a 20°-30° angle. Move bench away from attachment site to place desired tension level on tubing once in the starting position. Lie supine with head at high end and place feet on bench with knees bent.

B. Raise hands overhead, slightly wider than shoulders with palms facing each other. Have partner place a handle in each hand and bend elbows approximately 10°.

C. Keep wrists firm and arms in the starting position during the first one-third of the pull over motion while reaching toward the ceiling. During the next two-thirds of the motion, angle thumbs toward each other and focus on lifting the rib cage. Finish with the thumbs pointing at each other, hands over the lower chest, and arms fully straightened just inside shoulders.

D. Slowly return to the starting position without allowing the hips to raise.

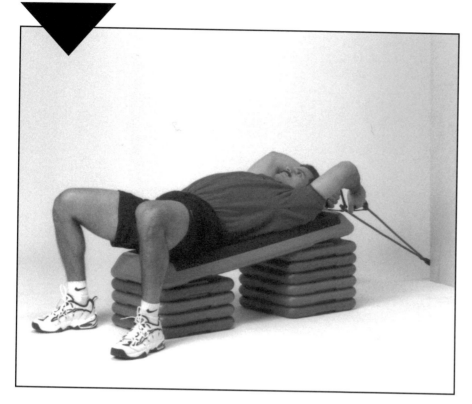

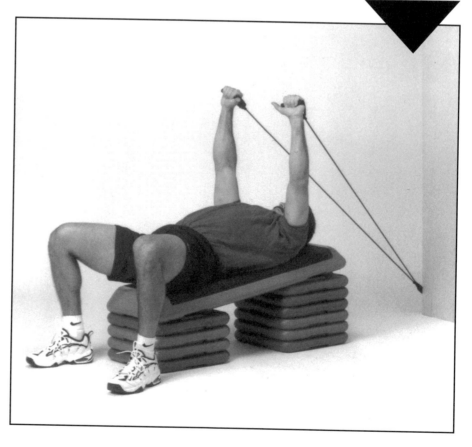

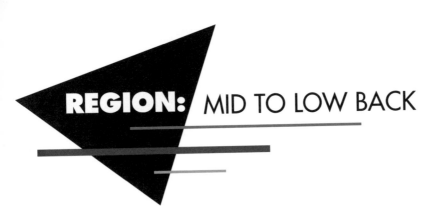

XERTUBE 20°-30° BENCH SUPINE STIFF ARM PULL OVER (HIGH ANCHOR)

(Latissimus Dorsi/Lower Trapezius)

A. Anchor tubing at top of door directly in line with middle of bench. Adjust end of bench closest to attachment site to a 20-30° angle. Move bench away from attachment site to place desired tension level on tubing once in the starting position. Lie supine with head at high end and place feet on bench with knees bent.

B. Raise hands overhead slightly wider than shoulders with palms facing up. Have partner place a handle in each hand with handles in the back portion of hands using a cupped grip.

C. Maintaining a stiff arm position, press downward keeping wrists firm and hands open while expanding the chest and lifting the rib cage. Finish with the shoulders fully extended, fingertips touching kneecaps, shoulder blades squeezed together, and bellybutton drawn toward spine.

D. Slowly return to the starting position without allowing the hips to raise.

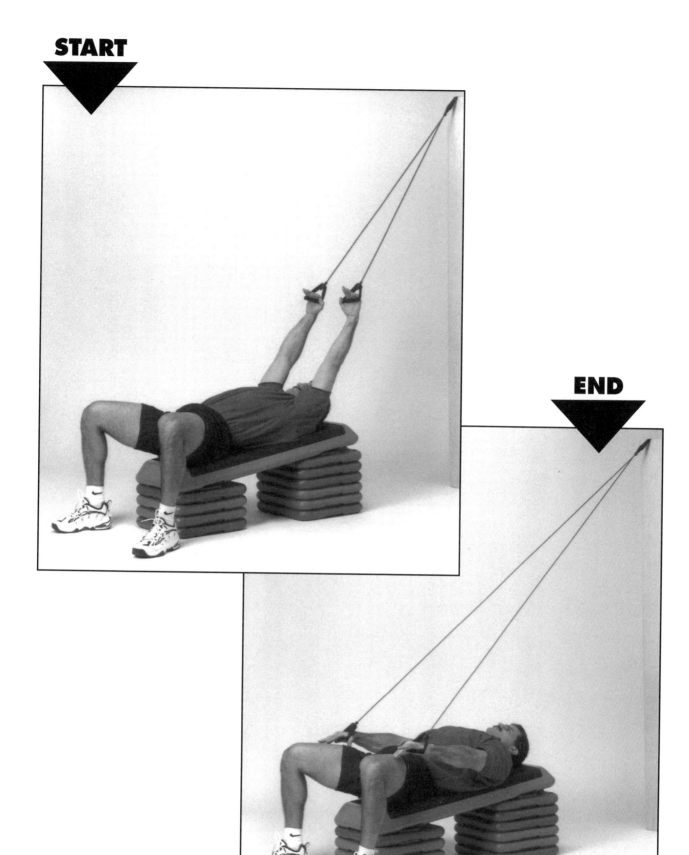

END

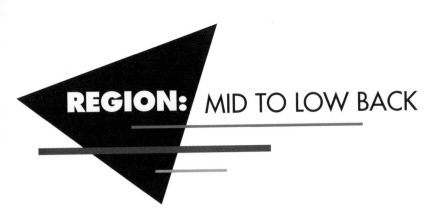

XERTUBE 20°-30° BENCH SUPINE BENT ARM PULL OVER (HIGH ANCHOR)

(Latissimus Dorsi/Lower Trapezius)

A. Anchor tubing at top of door directly in line with middle of bench. Adjust end of bench closest to attachment site to a 20°-30° angle. Move bench away from attachment site to place desired tension level on tubing once in the starting position. Lie supine with head at high end and place feet on bench with knees bent.

B. Raise hands overhead slightly wider than shoulders with palms facing each other. Have partner place a handle in each hand with palms facing each other and thumbs pointing down.

C. With firm wrists, lead with the elbows and upper arms driving them down toward the waistline. Progressively flare the elbows outward while expanding the chest and lifting the rib cage. Finish with the thumbs contacting the outer hips, arms bent, elbows flared, shoulder blades squeezed together, and bellybutton drawn toward spine (lat pose position).

D. Slowly return to the starting position without allowing the hips to raise.

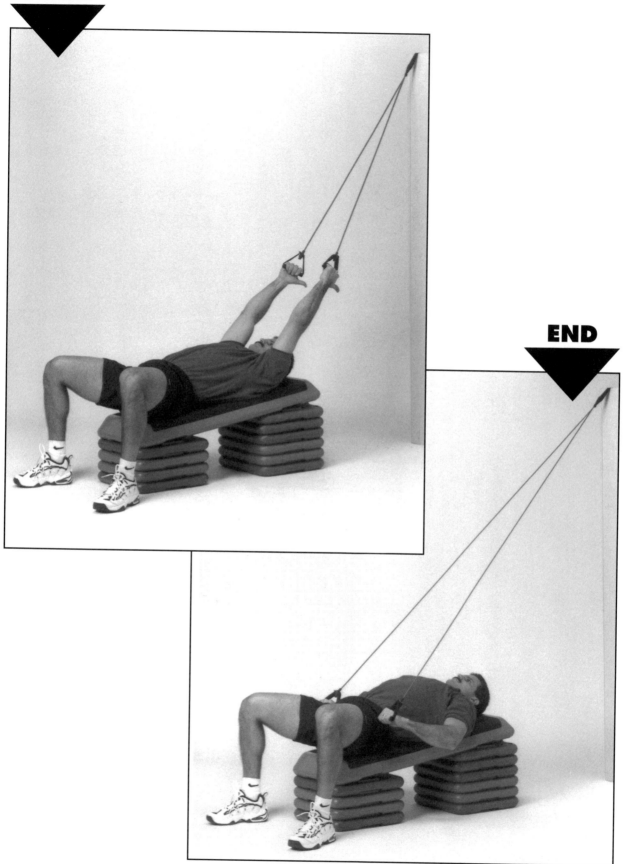

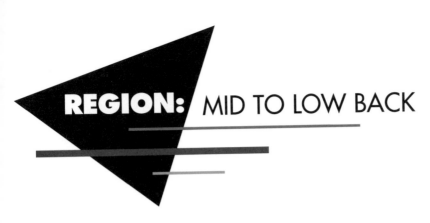
XERTUBE 20°-30° BENCH PRONE STIFF ARM PULL DOWN (HIGH ANCHOR)

(Latissimus Dorsi/Lower Trapezius)

A. Anchor tubing at top of door directly in line with middle of bench. Adjust end of bench closest to attachment site to a 20° to 30° angle. Move bench away from attachment site to place desired tension level on tubing once in the starting position. Lie prone with head at high end and place chin just over edge of bench. The knees should be bent comfortably with feet positioned just outside hip width and balls of feet on floor.

B. Have partner place a handle in each hand. Move handles to the back portion of hands and use a cupped grip.

C. Extend arms fully to shoulder height with palms facing down and eyes focusing down. Do not allow shoulders to elevate or shrug excessively. Keep the cervical spine neutral with eyes looking down at floor.

D. TWO ARM - Maintaining a stiff arm position, press downward keeping wrists firm and hands open while expanding the chest and lifting the rib cage. Finish with the shoulders fully extended, palms facing back and slightly outside hips, shoulder blades squeezed together, and bellybutton drawn toward spine. Slowly return to the starting position.

ALTERNATE ARMS - Using the same mechanics, press downward to the end position with one arm while keeping the other arm in the extended position. Then, simultaneously drive the arm in the extended position down while the opposite arm rises up. Continue this alternate arm motion for the desired number of repetitions.

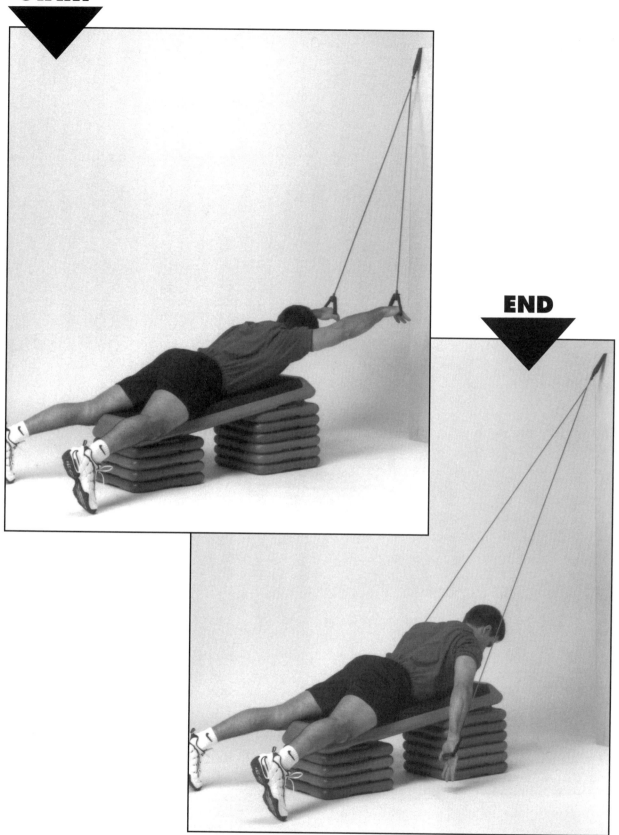

XERTUBE STANDING REVERSE PULL OVER
(Latissimus Dorsi/Lower Trapezius)

A. Anchor tubing at ankle height with torso facing attachment site.

B. Grasp a handle in each hand, move away from attachment site to desired tension level, and stand upright. Straighten arms toward floor at shoulder width, allowing arms to hang comfortably. The palms should face each other with thumbs up.

C. Place feet approximately shoulder width apart. Lead with hips and perform a half-squat while keeping arms straight. With firm wrists, pull up and back, keeping arms straight while simultaneously rising from the half-squat. Focus on expanding the chest, lifting the rib cage, and drawing the bellybutton toward spine.

D. Finish with the hands slightly wider than shoulders, arms straightened overhead, and thumbs pointing back. Keep the natural lumbar curvature while standing fully upright. Do not allow the pelvis to tuck under or the lower spine to arch excessively.

E. Slowly return to the half-squat starting position.

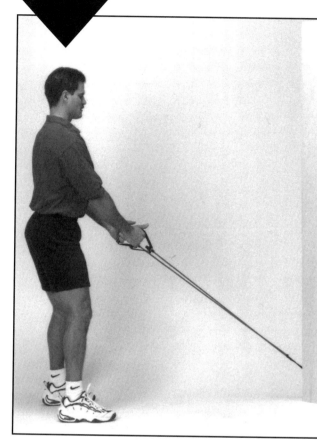

MID

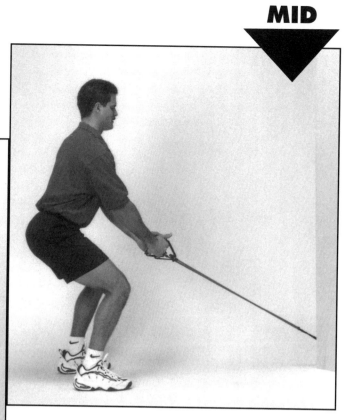

END

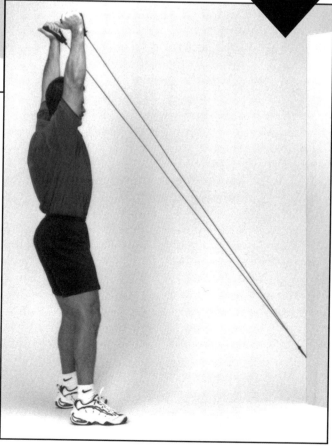

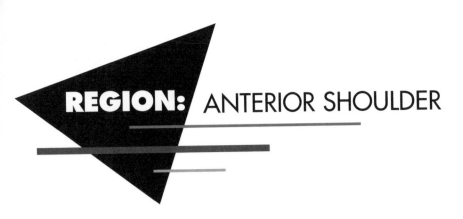

REGION: ANTERIOR SHOULDER

XERTUBE STANDING FRONT RAISE
(Anterior Deltoid/Lower Trapezius)

A. Stand in a staggered, narrow or wide stance. Place tubing under arch of front foot or both feet and soften knees. Keep hips back, tilt pelvis slightly anterior and lumbar spine neutral.

B. Grasp or rest backs of hands against handles. Place palms of hands against thighs with arms extended down directly under shoulders.

C. With firm wrists, lift arms up and forward. Gradually rotate in from shoulders slightly, leading with little fingers, as hands rise to shoulder height.

D. Finish with elbows soft and hands just outside shoulder width.

E. Keep the chest up, rib cage lifted, bellybutton drawn toward spine, and the lumbar spine in its neutral curvature.

> ## TECH TIPS
> **This exercise may be performed on one side only by standing on one end of tubing.**

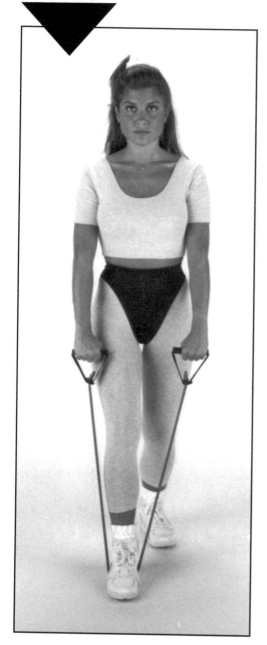

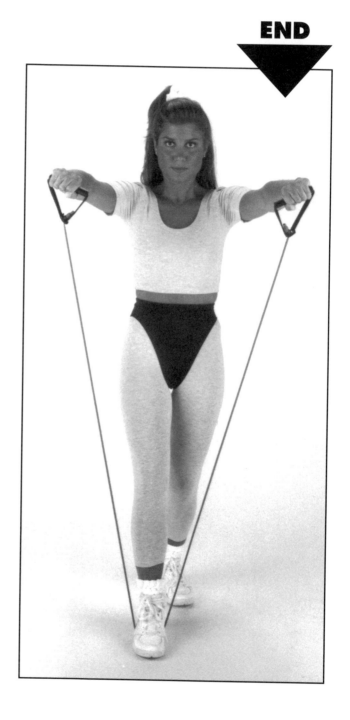

STEP XERTUBE STANDING FRONT RAISE

(Anterior Deltoid)

A. Tubing is secured through step strap at outside attachment.

B. Grasp handles and stand on step in a narrow, staggered lunge position nearest to step strap. Soften knees, keep hips back, tilt pelvis slightly anterior and lumbar spine neutral.

C. Grasp or rest backs of hands against handles. Place palms of hands against thighs with arms extended down directly under shoulders.

D. With firm wrists, lift arms up and forward. Gradually rotate in from shoulders slightly, leading with little fingers as hands rise to shoulder height.

E. Finish with elbows soft and hands just outside shoulder width.

F. Keep the chest up, rib cage lifted, bellybutton drawn toward spine, and the lumbar spine in its neutral curvature.

TECH TIPS

This exercise may be performed one side at a time.

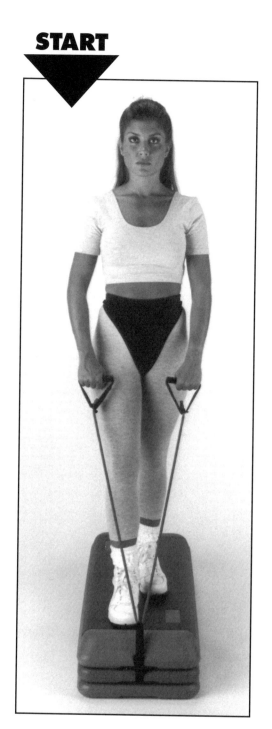

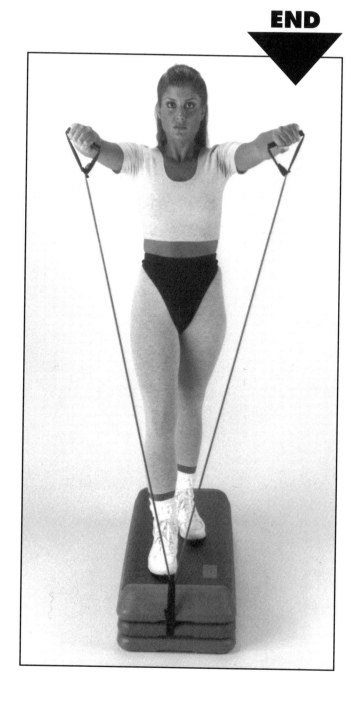

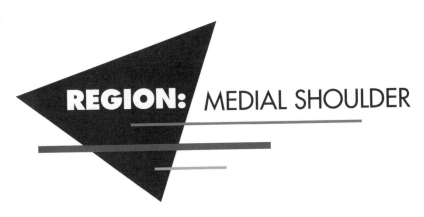

REGION: MEDIAL SHOULDER

XERTUBE STANDING SIDE RAISE (STRAIGHT ARM/BENT ARM)

(Medial Deltoid)

A. Stand in a staggered, narrow or wide stance. Place tubing under arch of front foot or both feet, and soften knees. Keep hips back, tilt pelvis slightly anterior and lumbar spine neutral.

B. Grasp handles, maintain a slight bend in elbows and position arms straight down from shoulders with thumbs pointing forward.

C. STRAIGHT ARM - With firm wrists, lift arms up and away from sides of body. Progressively rotate shoulders back as elbows rise to shoulder height.

BENT ARM - Bend and flare elbows and immediately face palms toward floor. Hands are kept at elbow height as they are moved away from sides of body. Upper and lower arms move as one unit and wrists remain firm.

D. STRAIGHT ARM - Finish with thumbs up and palms facing forward, elbows soft and in alignment with shoulder joint. Hands should be just in front of ears.

BENT ARM - Elbows should be at same height as hands and parallel to shoulders. End with upper and lower arms forming 90° angles.

E. Keep the chest up, rib cage lifted, bellybutton drawn toward spine, and the lumbar spine in its neutral curvature.

TECH TIPS

This exercise may be performed on one side by standing on one end of tubing.

This exercise may also be performed by anchoring tubing at ankle height. Turn so non-exercising shoulder is parallel to and nearest to attachment. Exercising arm will start at midline of body. Assume a square stance and with a single arm, perform steps C through E.

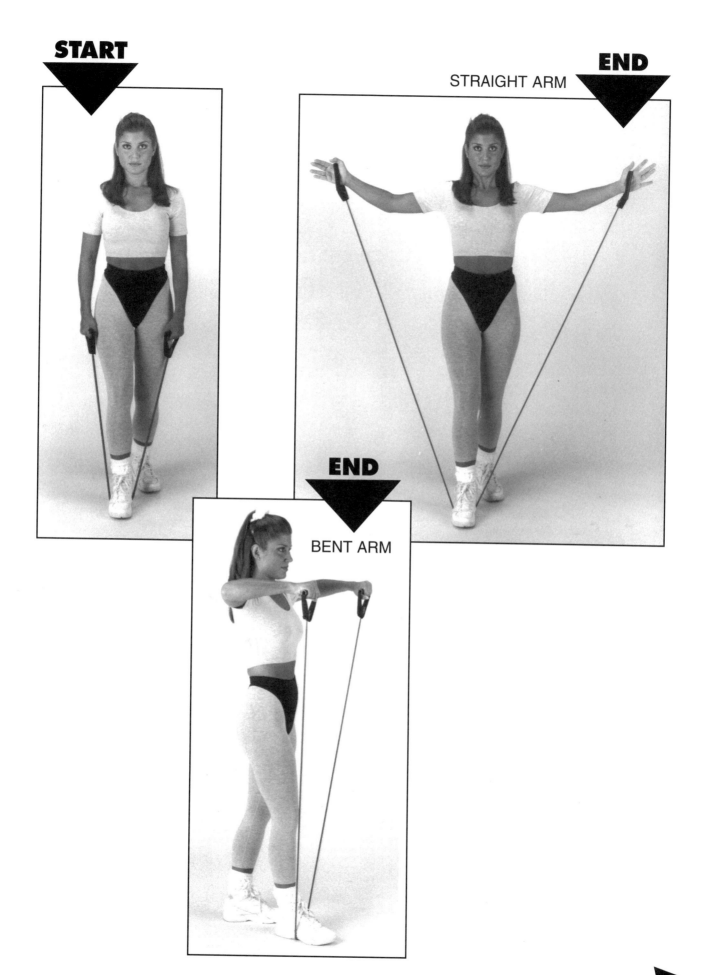

START

STRAIGHT ARM **END**

END

BENT ARM

XERTUBE STANDING SINGLE ARM BENT ARM SIDE RAISE TO EXTERNAL ROTATION

(Medial Deltoid, External Rotators)

▼ End position of shoulder joint - 90° Abduction

A. Anchor tubing at ankle height and position torso parallel to and behind attachment site approximately 12".

B. Grasp handle(s) in hand furthest from attachment site and place opposite hand on hip. Move away from attachment site to desired tension level and assume a quarter-squat position. Keep hips back, pelvis tilted slightly anterior, lumbar spine neutral and torso slightly forward (athletic position). Keep torso square with palm of exercising hand slightly in front of opposite hip with thumb up and upper and lower arm at a 90° angle.

C. With a firm wrist, lead with upper arm and abduct shoulder to 90° so that the elbow is parallel to shoulder with palm down (phase 1). Maintain the upper and lower arm angle with chest expanded, rib cage lifted, and belly button drawn toward spine.

D. Immediately as the elbow reaches shoulder height, externally rotate the shoulder performing a semicircular motion with the lower arm. The upper arm, elbow, and torso must remain stationary. The quarter-squat athletic position must be maintained.

E. Finish with knuckles facing ceiling and palm facing forward.

F. Slowly return to the starting position. Turn body the opposite direction and repeat an equal amount of repetitions.

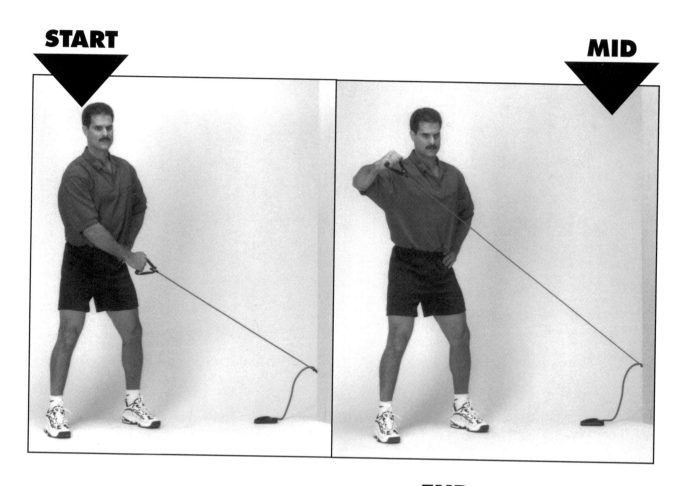

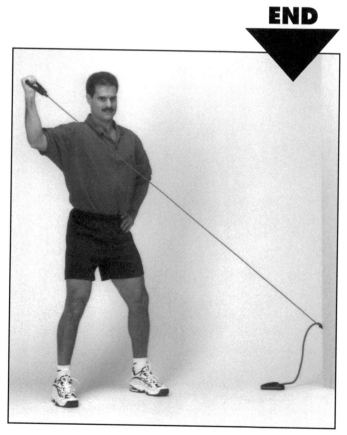

XERTUBE STANDING REVERSE FLYE
(High Pull or Low Pull)

(Posterior Deltoid)

A. Anchor tubing at shoulder height, grasp or place backs of open hands against handles with thumbs up. Back away from insertion until arms fully lengthen.

B. Assume a staggered lunge position and soften knees. Keep hips back, tilt pelvis slightly anterior and lumbar spine neutral.

C. **HIGH PULL -** With firm wrists and a slight bend in elbows, pull back until shoulder blades are squeezed together.

  LOW PULL - With firm wrists pull down and back and gradually rotate shoulders back so palms face away from body.

D. **HIGH PULL -** Hands end parallel to, and slightly behind shoulders in a thumbs up position.

  LOW PULL - Hands end behind body with shoulders fully extended and equal to height of hips.

E. Keep the chest up, rib cage lifted, bellybutton drawn toward spine, and the lumbar spine in its neutral curvature.

TECH TIPS
The joint function of horizontal shoulder abduction recruits the posterior deltoid during the high pull. The joint function of shoulder extension recruits the posterior deltoid during the low pull.

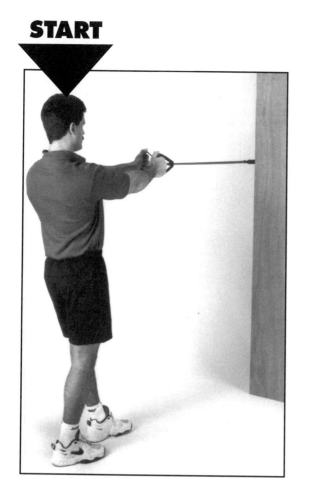

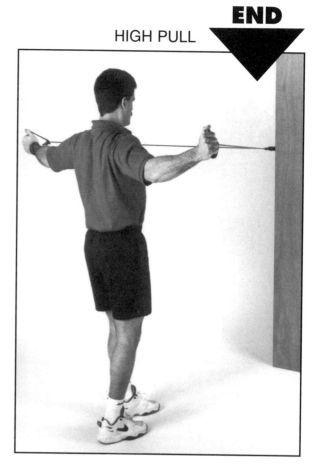

LOW PULL **END**

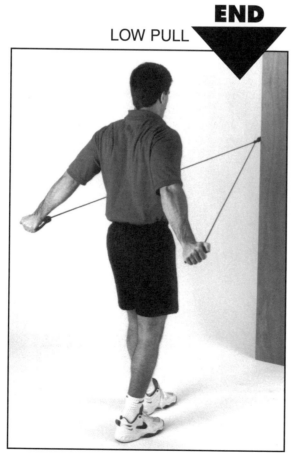

XERTUBE PARTNER STANDING REVERSE FLYE
(Posterior Deltoid, Rhomboids, Middle Trapezius)

A. Exerciser stands facing partner. Two Xertubes are used simultaneously for this exercise. Each person grasps one handle of the same Xertube with the right hand and one handle of the other Xertube with the left. Switch handles in hands making an X pattern with the Xertubes.

B. Move away from each other taking steps backward to a desired tension level and assume a quarter-squat position. Keep hips back, pelvis tilted slightly, lumbar spine neutral, and lean torso forward slightly (athletic position). Extend arms fully at shoulder height with palms facing each other.

C. With firm wrists and soft elbows (5° bend), pull out and back while expanding the chest, lifting the rib cage, and drawing the bellybutton toward spine.

D. Finish with hands parallel to and slightly behind shoulders in a thumbs up position and shoulder blades squeezed together. The quarter-squat athletic position must be maintained throughout.

E. Slowly return to the starting position.

START

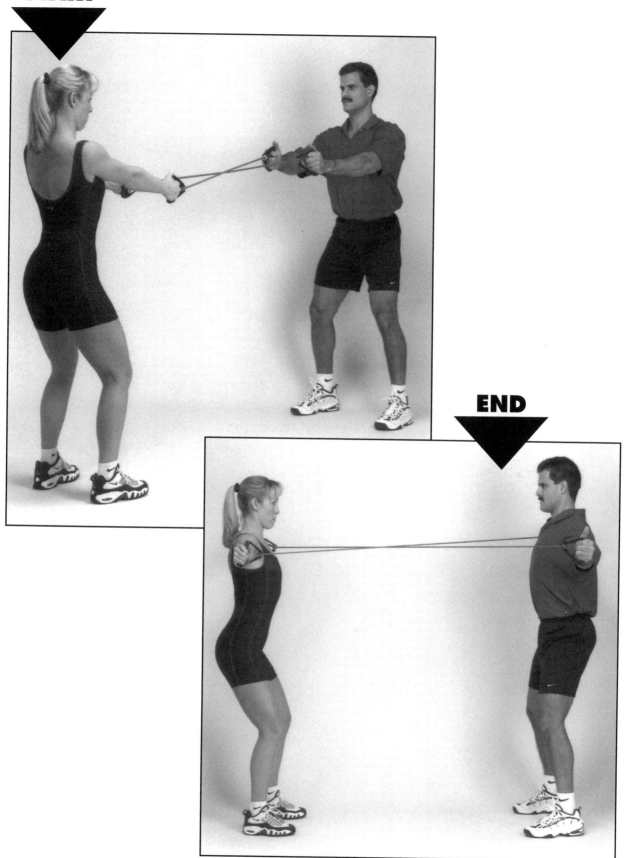

END

XERTUBE STANDING SINGLE ARM REVERSE FLYE
(Posterior Deltoid, Rhomboids, Middle Trapezius)

A. Anchor tubing at shoulder height when standing. Position torso parallel to and slightly behind attachment site approximately 12".

B. Grasp handle in hand furthest from attachment site. Move away from attachment site to desired tension level and assume a quarter-squat position. Keep hips back, pelvis tilted slightly anterior, lumber spine neutral, and torso slightly forward (athletic position). Keep torso square with elbow bent and shoulder adducted comfortably across body at shoulder height. The knuckles should face the attachment site. Place the non-involved hand on hip.

C. With wrist firm, pull out and away from body progressively straightening arm. Keep the chest expanded, rib cage lifted, and bellybutton drawn toward spine.

D. Finish with hand parallel to shoulder, arm straightened with palm facing forward, and shoulder blade squeezed toward spine. The tubing should end resting against the upper chest. The quarter-squat athletic position must be maintained.

E. Slowly return to the starting position. Turn the opposite direction and repeat an equal amount of repetitions.

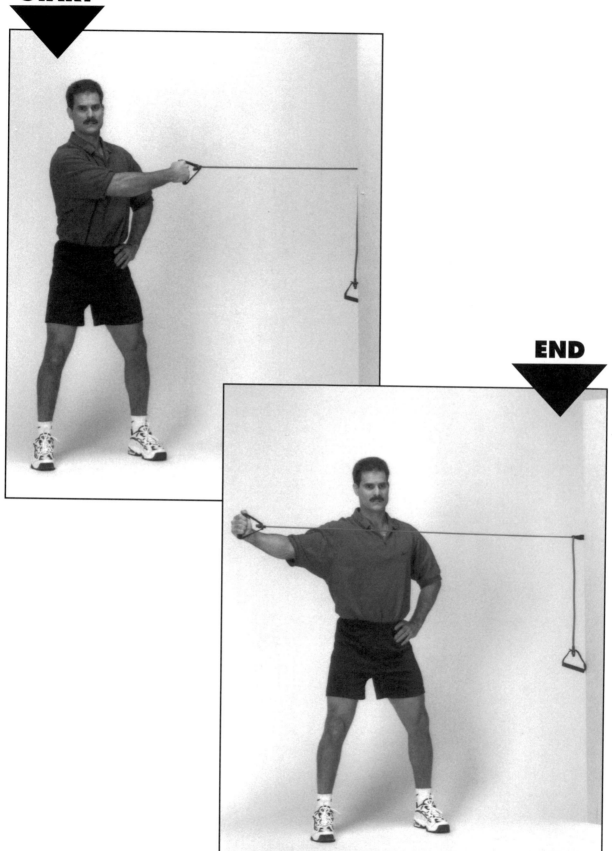

XERTUBE PARTNER STANDING SINGLE ARM REVERSE FLYE

(Posterior Deltoid, Rhomboids, Middle Trapezius)

A. Exerciser and partner stand next to each other and align right shoulders. Each person grasps one handle with the left hand.

B. Move away from each other taking steps laterally to a desired tension level and assume a quarter-squat position. Keep hips back, pelvis tilted slightly anterior, lumbar spine neutral, and torso slightly forward (athletic position). Keep torso square with elbow bent and shoulder adducted comfortably across body at shoulder height. The knuckles should face the attachment site. Place the uninvolved hand on hip.

C. With wrist firm, pull out and away from body gradually straightening arm. Keep the chest expanded, rib cage lifted, and bellybutton drawn toward spine.

D. Finish with hand parallel to shoulder, arm straightened with palm facing forward, and shoulder blade squeezed toward spine. The tubing should end resting against the upper chest. The quarter-squat athletic position must be maintained.

E. Slowly return to the starting position. Turn the opposite direction and repeat an equal amount of repetitions.

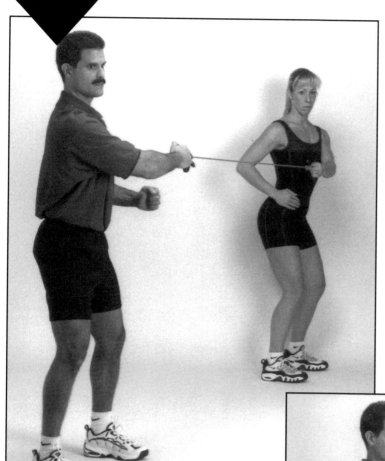

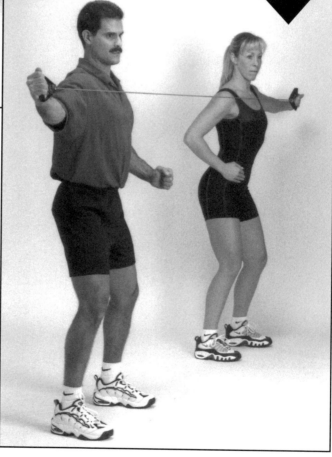

XERTUBE STANDING SINGLE ARM D1 PATTERN (Diagonal Backhand)

(Posterior Deltoid)

A. Anchor tubing at top of door when standing. Position torso parallel to and behind attachment site approximately 12".

B. Grasp handle(s) in hand furthest from attachment site and place opposite hand on hip. Move away from attachment site to desired tension level and assume a quarter-squat position. Keep hips back, pelvis tilted slightly anterior, lumbar spine neutral, and torso slightly forward (athletic position). Keep torso square and reach across body toward insertion with palm of hand facing front of shoulder nearest to attachment site. Do not elevate or shrug shoulder.

C. With a firm wrist, pull diagonally down gradually straightening arm. Keep the chest expanded, rib cage lifted, and bellybutton drawn toward spine.

D. Finish with palm facing forward parallel to hip, with shoulder abducted approximately 30° and shoulder blade squeezed toward spine. The quarter-squat athletic position must be maintained.

E. Slowly return to the starting position. Turn body the opposite direction and repeat an equal amount of repetitions.

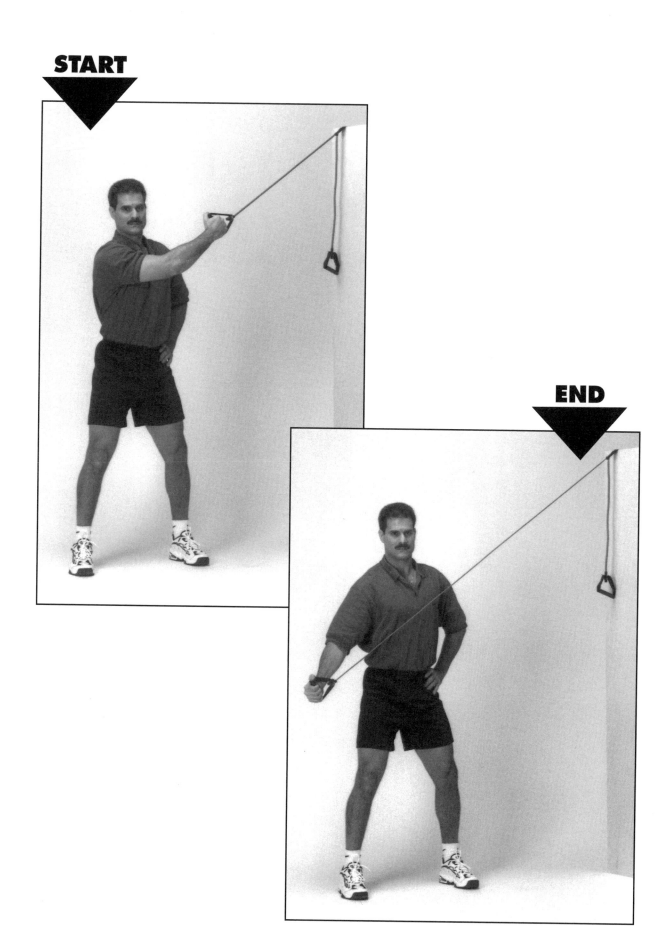

XERTUBE BENT OVER SINGLE ARM REVERSE FLYE

(Posterior Deltoid)

A. Anchor tubing at ankle height.

B. Grasp handles and turn so your non-exercising shoulder is parallel with and nearest to attachment.

C. Position feet slightly wider than shoulder width, bend over so chest is approximately parallel to floor, and assume a half-squat position.

D. Position exercising hand in a palm up position and place other hand on your opposite thigh.

E. With firm wrist, pull up and out across body. The hand will progress to a palm down position as arm fully extends out from shoulder. Shoulders must stay square.

F. Keep the chest up, rib cage lifted, bellybutton drawn toward spine, and the lumbar spine in its neutral curvature.

G. Turn the opposite direction and repeat equal amounts of repetitions with other hand.

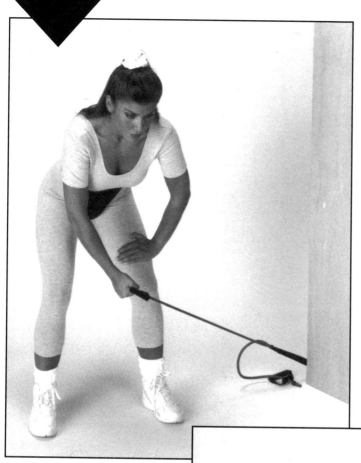

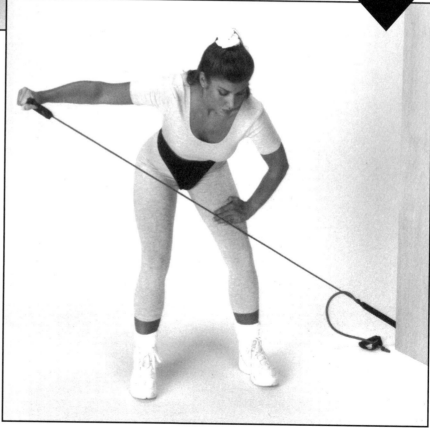

STEP XERTUBE   BENT OVER SINGLE ARM REVERSE FLYE

(Posterior Deltoid)

A. Tubing is secured through step strap at outside attachment. Stand at end of step furthest away from step strap.

B. Turn so your non-exercising shoulder is parallel with and nearest to attachment.

C. Place the foot nearest to step directly over middle of step block and other foot on floor. For safety, use only one block under each end of step. Grasp handle with hand furthest from attachment site.

D. Position feet slightly wider than shoulder width, bend over so chest is approximately parallel to floor, and assume a half-squat position.

E. Position exercising hand in a palm up position and place other hand on your opposite thigh.

F. With firm wrist, pull up and out across body. The hand will progress to a palm down position as arm fully extends out from shoulder. Shoulders must stay square.

G. Keep the chest up, rib cage lifted, bellybutton drawn toward spine, and the lumbar spine in its neutral curvature.

H. Turn the opposite direction and repeat equal amounts of repetitions with other hand.

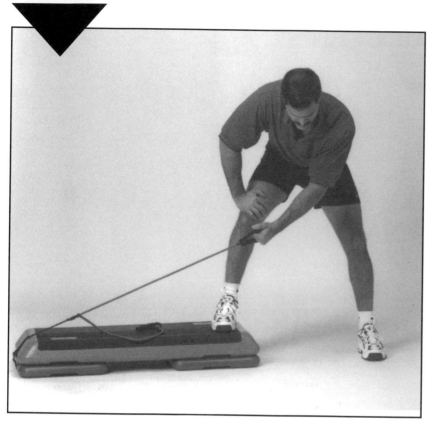

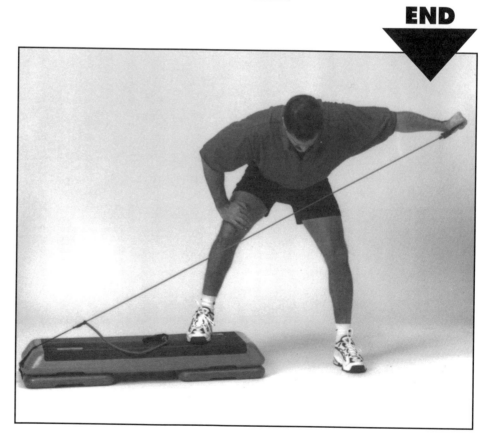

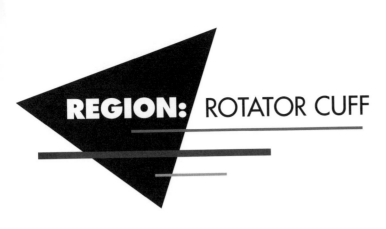

XERTUBE STANDING EXTERNAL SHOULDER ROTATION

(External Rotators)

▼ **Position of shoulder joint - 0° to 20° Abduction (neutral position)**

A. Stand in a square or staggered stance. Anchor tubing at waist height and soften knees. Keep hips back, tilt pelvis slightly anterior and lumbar spine neutral.

B. Grasp handle with exercising hand and turn so non-exercising arm is parallel with and nearest to attachment. Place palm of exercising hand against torso at level of navel and point thumb upward (internal shoulder rotation).

C. Keep elbow flexed 90° directly under shoulder (neutral position). With a firm wrist, gradually rotate shoulder outward by pulling tubing away from body, performing a semicircular motion with lower arm.

D. Finish with thumb pointing upward, elbow directly under shoulder and shoulder rotated out through its full range of motion.

E. Keep the chest up, rib cage lifted, bellybutton drawn toward spine and the lumbar spine in its neutral curvature.

F. Turn the opposite direction and repeat equal amounts of repetitions with other hand.

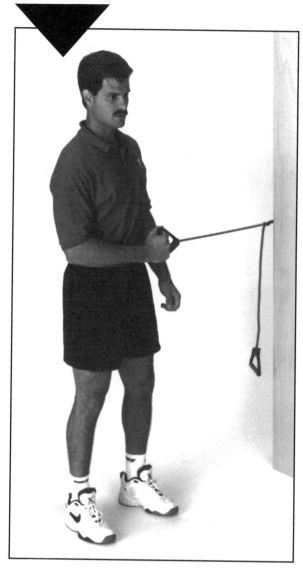

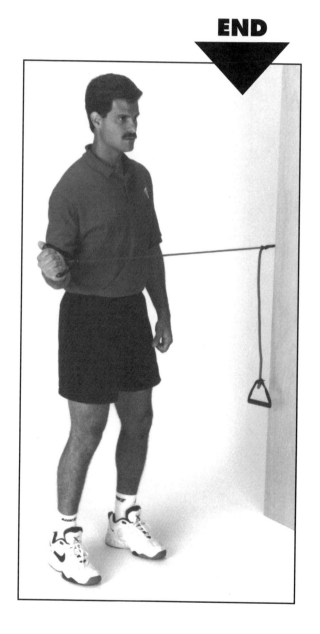

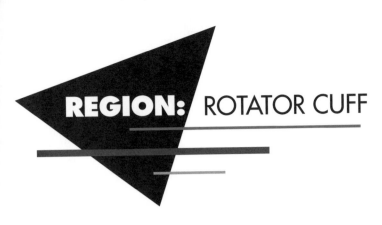

REGION: ROTATOR CUFF

XERTUBE PARTNER STANDING EXTERNAL SHOULDER ROTATION

(External Rotators)

▼ **Position of shoulder joint - 0° to 20° Abduction (neutral position)**

A. Exerciser and partner stand next to each other and align right shoulders. Each person grasps one handle with the left hand.

B. Move away from each other taking steps laterally to a desired tension level and assume a quarter-squat position. Keep hips back, pelvis tilted slightly anterior, lumbar spine neutral and torso slightly forward (athletic position). Position palm of exercising hand in front of navel with thumb up and upper and lower arm bent 90° (shoulder internal rotation). Keep the elbow directly under or slightly outside shoulder. Place opposite hand on hip.

C. With a firm wrist, externally rotate shoulder performing a semicircular motion with the lower arm. The upper arm, elbow and torso must remain stationary. Keep the chest expanded, rib cage lifted and bellybutton drawn toward spine. The quarter-squat athletic position must be maintained.

D. Finish with the elbow in the same starting position and shoulder externally rotated through its full range of motion with palm facing forward.

E. Slowly return to the starting position. Turn body the opposite direction and repeat an equal amount of repetitions.

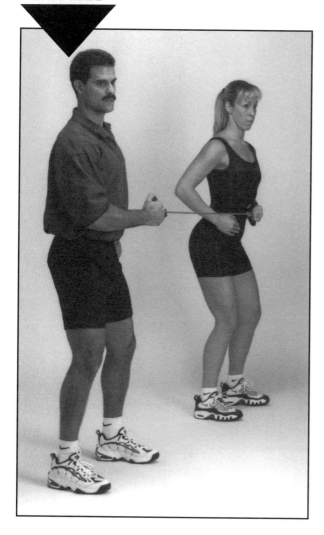

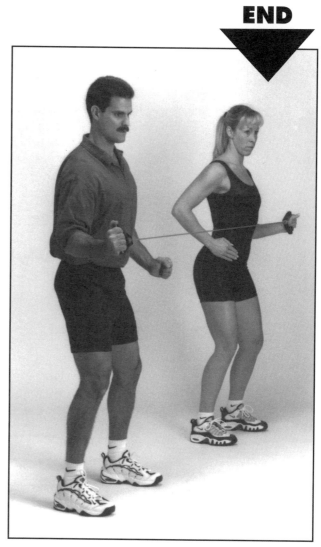

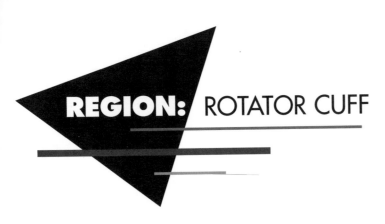

XERTUBE STANDING EXTERNAL SHOULDER ROTATION

(External Rotators)

▼ **Position of shoulder joint - 70° Abduction, 30° Flexion**

A. Stand in a square or staggered stance. Anchor tubing between knee and waist height and soften knees. Keep hips back, tilt pelvis slightly anterior and lumbar spine neutral.

B. Grasp handle with exercising hand and turn so non-exercising arm is parallel with and nearest to attachment. Abduct arm 70° and flex 30°, face palm downward and point thumb toward lower chest (internal shoulder rotation).

C. With a firm wrist, gradually rotate shoulder outward by pulling tubing away from body performing a semicircular motion with lower arm.

D. Finish with thumb pointing backward, elbow in same position as above, and shoulder rotated out through its full range of motion.

E. Keep the chest up, rib cage lifted, bellybutton drawn toward spine and the lumbar spine in its neutral curvature.

F. Turn the opposite direction and repeat equal amounts of repetitions with other hand.

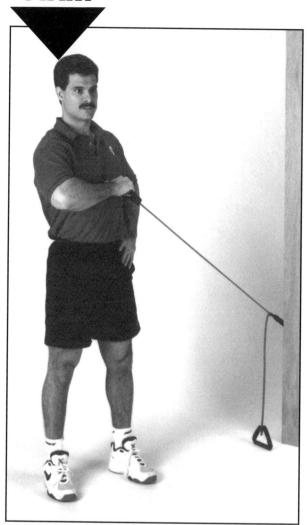

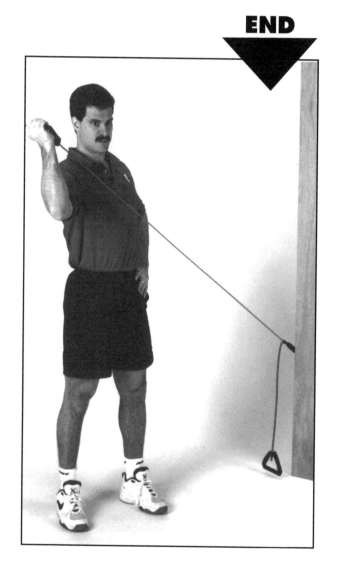

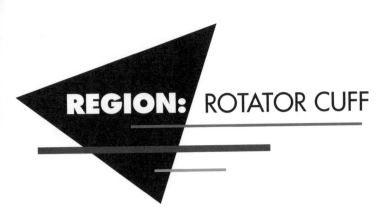

XERTUBE STANDING EXTERNAL SHOULDER ROTATION

(External Rotators)

▼ **Position of shoulder joint - 90° Abduction**

A. Stand in a square or staggered stance. Anchor tubing between knee and waist height and soften knees. Keep hips back, tilt pelvis slightly anterior and lumbar spine neutral.

B. Grasp handle with exercising hand and face attachment site. Abduct arm 90°, face palm downward and point thumb toward midline of body (internal rotation).

C. With a firm wrist, gradually rotate shoulder back by pulling tubing back with a semicircular motion of lower arm.

D. Finish with thumb pointing toward midline of body, elbow in same position as above, and shoulder rotated back through its full range of motion.

E. Keep the chest up, rib cage lifted, bellybutton drawn toward spine and the lumbar spine in its neutral curvature.

F. Align the other shoulder with the attachment site and repeat equal amounts of repetitions with other hand.

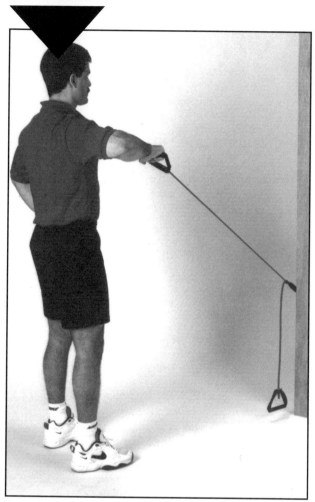

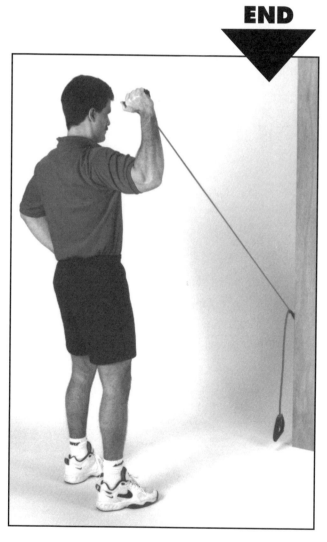

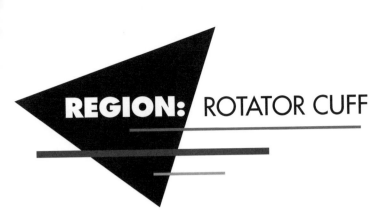

XERTUBE PARTNER STANDING EXTERNAL SHOULDER ROTATION

(External Rotators)

▼ Position of shoulder joint - 90° Abduction

A. Exerciser and partner stand facing each other. Each person grasps one handle with the same hand.

B. Move away from each other taking steps backward to a desired tension level and assume a quarter-squat position. Keep hips back, pelvis tilted slightly anterior, lumbar spine neutral, and lean torso forward slightly (athletic position). Extend arm fully at shoulder height with palm facing down.

C. Pull back so that elbow stops parallel to shoulder. The shoulder should be abducted 90° with the upper and lower arm forming a 90° angle (internal rotation). Do not allow the shoulder to shrug or elevate. The tubing should form a straight line from hand to hand.

D. With a firm wrist, externally rotate shoulder performing a semicircular motion with the lower arm. The upper arm, elbow and torso must remain stationary. Keep the chest expanded, rib cage lifted, and bellybutton drawn toward spine.

E. Finish with the elbow in the same starting position and shoulder externally rotated through its full range of motion with palm facing forward and knuckles at ceiling. The quarter-squat athletic position must be maintained throughout.

F. Slowly return to the starting position. Place handle in opposite hand and repeat an equal amount of repetitions.

START

END

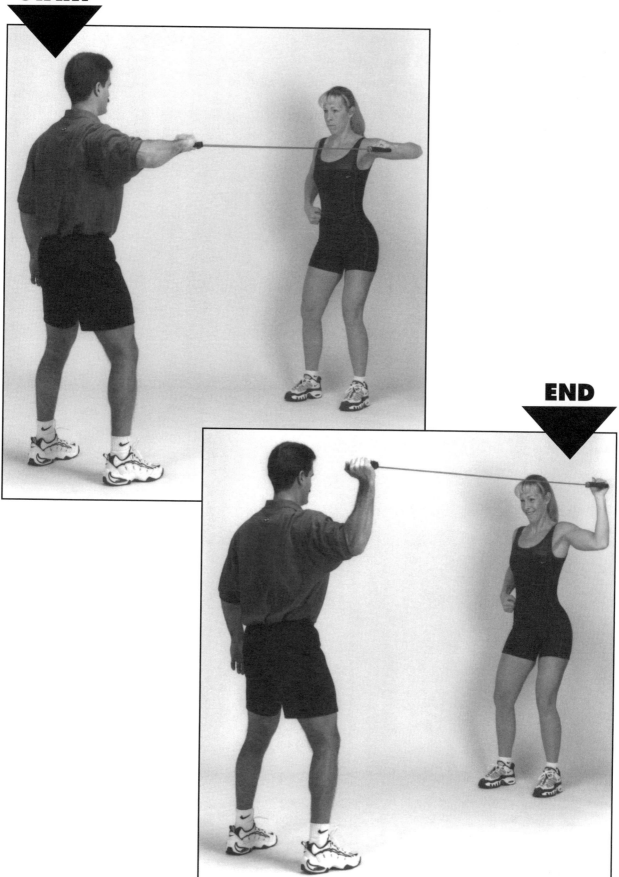

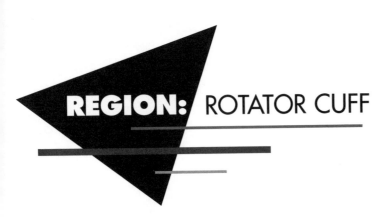

XERTUBE STANDING D2 PATTERN
(Medial Shoulder/External Rotators)

A. Anchor tubing at ankle height and stand in a square stance. Assume a quarter-squat position, keep hips back, tilt pelvis slightly anterior and lumbar spine neutral.

B. Grasp handle with exercising hand and turn so non-exercising arm is parallel with and nearest to attachment. Begin with thumb placed against hip of uninvolved side of body (internal shoulder rotation).

C. With a firm wrist, gradually rotate shoulder outward by pulling tubing upward and across the body in a sweeping arc.

D. Finish with thumb pointing behind body, shoulder abducted 80-85° and shoulder rotated out through its full range of motion.

E. Keep the chest up, rib cage lifted, bellybutton drawn toward spine and the lumbar spine in its neutral curvature.

F. Turn the opposite direction and repeat equal amounts of repetitions with other hand.

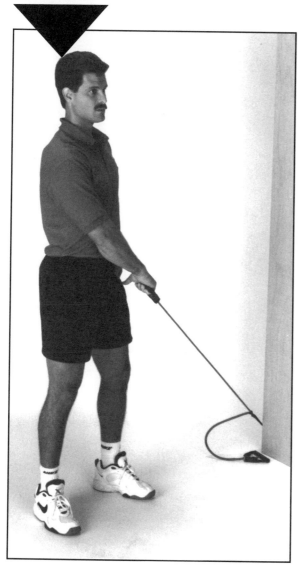

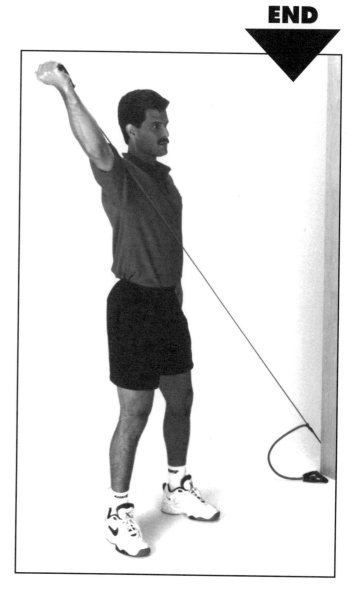

THE COMPLETE GUIDE TO **RUBBERIZED RESISTANCE EXERCISES** 113

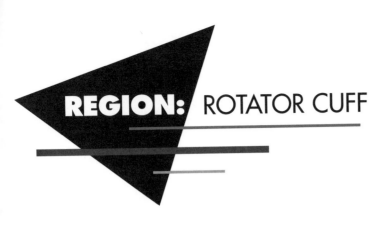

STEP XERTUBE STANDING SINGLE ARM D2 PATTERN

(Medial Deltoid/External Rotators)

A. Stand at end of step farthest away from step strap.

B. Tubing is secured through step strap at outside attachment.

C. Turn so non-exercising arm is parallel with and nearest to attachment. Straighten both arms directly under shoulders.

D. Place the foot nearest to step directly over middle of step block and other foot on floor. For safety, use only one block under each end of step. Grasp handle in hand furthest away from attachment site and assume a quarter-squat position. Keep hips back, tilt pelvis slightly anterior and lumbar spine neutral.

E. With firm wrist, lift exercising arm up and away from side of body, keeping arm as straight as possible. Gradually rotate shoulder back as elbow raises to shoulder height.

F. Finish with thumb up and palm facing forward, elbow soft and in alignment with shoulder joint. Hand should be just above shoulder height.

G. Keep the chest up, rib cage lifted, bellybutton drawn toward spine and the lumbar spine in its neutral curvature.

H. Turn the opposite direction and repeat equal amounts of repetitions with other hand.

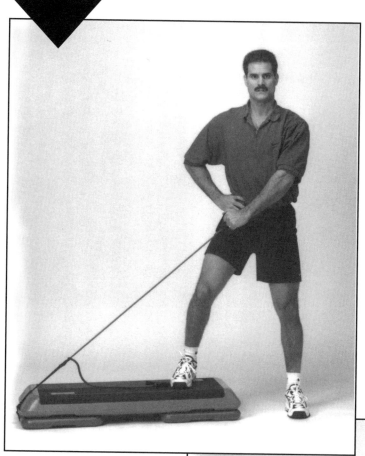

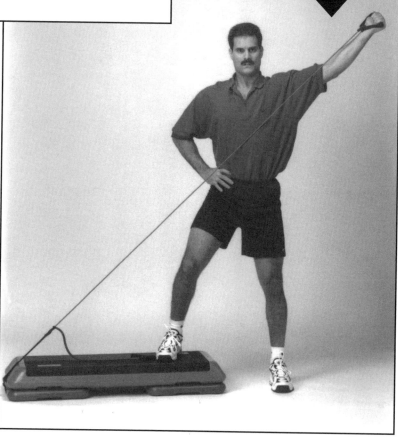

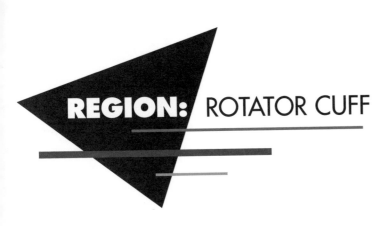

XERTUBE STANDING INTERNAL SHOULDER ROTATION

(Internal Rotators)

▼ Position of shoulder joint - 0°-20° Abduction

A. Stand in a square or staggered stance. Anchor tubing at waist height and soften knees. Keep hips back, tilt pelvis slightly anterior and lumbar spine neutral.

B. Grasp handle with exercising hand and turn so exercising arm is parallel with and nearest to attachment. Position elbow directly under shoulder (90° elbow flexion), turn shoulder outward away from body (external shoulder rotation), face palm forward and point thumb upward.

C. Keep elbow directly underneath shoulder, (neutral position). With a firm wrist, gradually rotate shoulder inward by pulling tubing toward torso, performing a semicircular motion with lower arm.

D. Finish with thumb pointing upward, palm against torso at level of navel, and shoulder rotated inward through its full range of motion.

E. Keep the chest up, rib cage lifted, bellybutton drawn toward spine and the lumbar spine in its neutral curvature.

F. Turn the opposite direction and repeat equal amounts of repetitions with other hand.

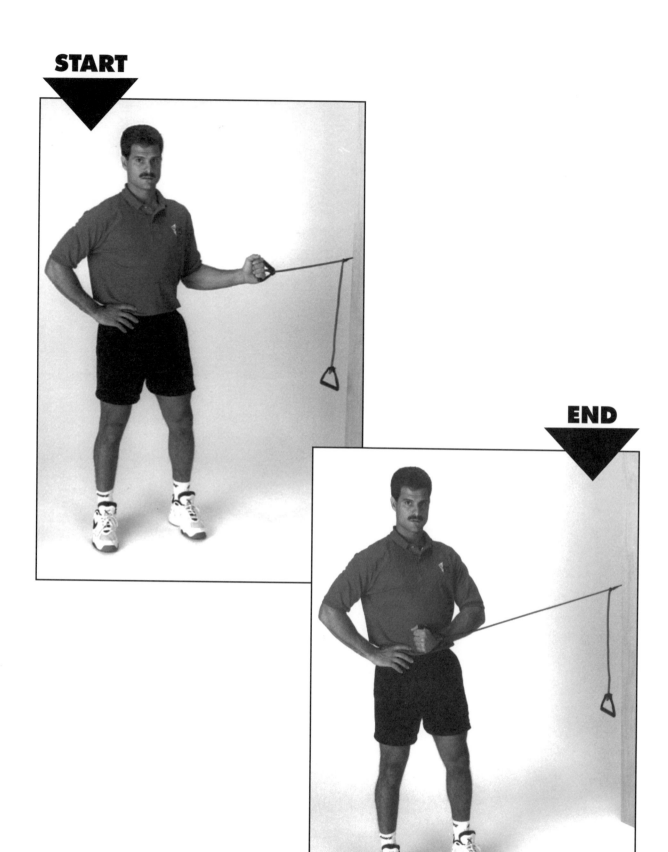

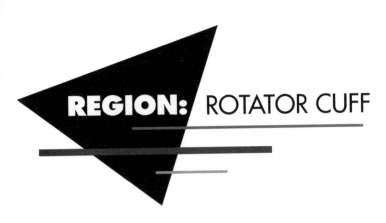

REGION: ROTATOR CUFF

XERTUBE STANDING INTERNAL SHOULDER ROTATION

(Internal Rotators)

▼ **Position of shoulder joint - 70° Abduction, 30° Flexion**

A. Stand in a square or staggered stance. Anchor tubing just above shoulder height and soften knees. Keep hips back, tilt pelvis slightly anterior and lumbar spine neutral.

B. Grasp handle with exercising hand and turn so exercising arm is parallel with and nearest to attachment. Abduct arm 70° and flex 30°, face palm forward and point thumb behind body (external shoulder rotation).

C. With a firm wrist, gradually rotate shoulder inward by pulling tubing in with a semi-circular motion of lower arm.

D. Finish with thumb pointing toward midline of body between navel and lower sternum, elbow in same position above, and shoulder rotated inward through its full range of motion.

E. Keep the chest up, rib cage lifted, bellybutton drawn toward spine and the lumbar spine in its neutral curvature.

F. Turn the opposite direction and repeat equal amounts of repetitions with other hand.

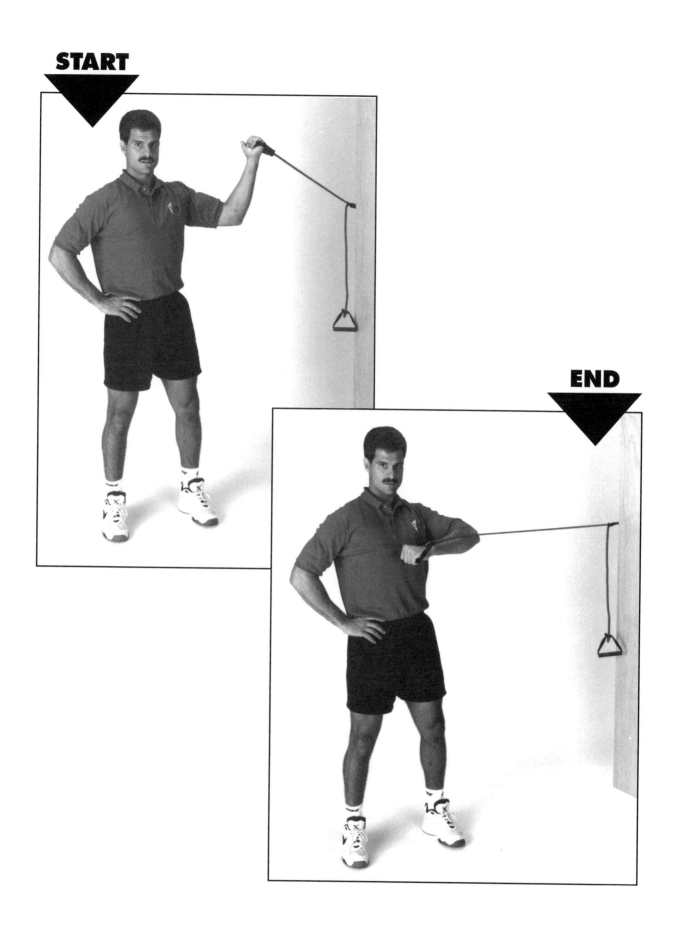

START

END

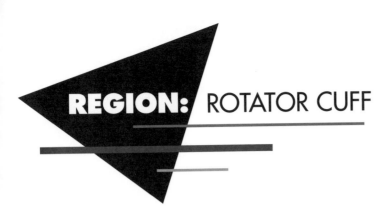

REGION: ROTATOR CUFF

XERTUBE STANDING INTERNAL SHOULDER ROTATION

(Internal Rotators)

▼ **Position of shoulder joint - 90° Abduction**

A. Stand in a square or staggered stance. Anchor tubing just above shoulder height and soften knees. Keep hips back, tilt pelvis slightly anterior and lumbar spine neutral.

B. Grasp handle with exercising hand and face away from attachment site. Abduct arm 90°, face palm forward and point thumb toward ear (external shoulder rotation).

C. With a firm wrist, gradually rotate shoulder in by pulling tubing down with a semicircular motion of lower arm.

D. Finish with thumb pointing toward midline of body, palm down, elbow in same position as above, and shoulder rotated inward through its full range of motion.

E. Keep the chest up, rib cage lifted, bellybutton drawn toward spine and the lumbar spine in its neutral curvature.

F. Align the other shoulder with the attachment site and repeat equal amounts of repetitions with other hand.

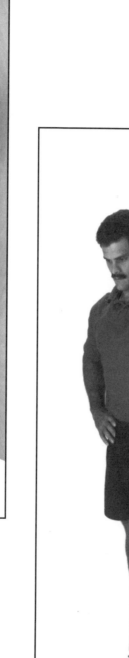

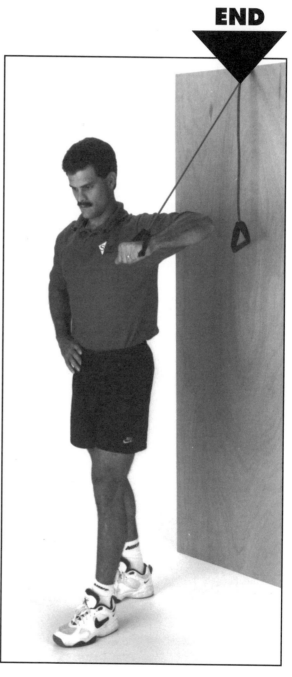

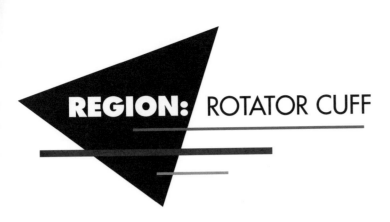

XERTUBE STANDING REVERSE D2 PATTERN

(Internal Rotators/Pectorals)

A. Stand in a square or staggered stance with hips back, pelvis tilted slightly anterior and lumbar spine neutral. Anchor tubing above head level. Turn so exercising arm is parallel to and just in front of tubing insertion with arm slightly above and behind shoulder.

B. Grasp handle with shoulder abducted approximately 90° and thumb pointing behind body (external shoulder rotation).

C. With a firm wrist, gradually rotate shoulder inward by pulling tubing downward and across the body in a sweeping arc.

D. Finish with thumb touching opposite hip, and shoulder rotated inward through its full range of motion.

E. Keep the chest up, rib cage lifted, bellybutton drawn toward spine and the lumbar spine in its neutral curvature.

F. Turn the opposite direction and repeat equal amounts of repetitions with other hand.

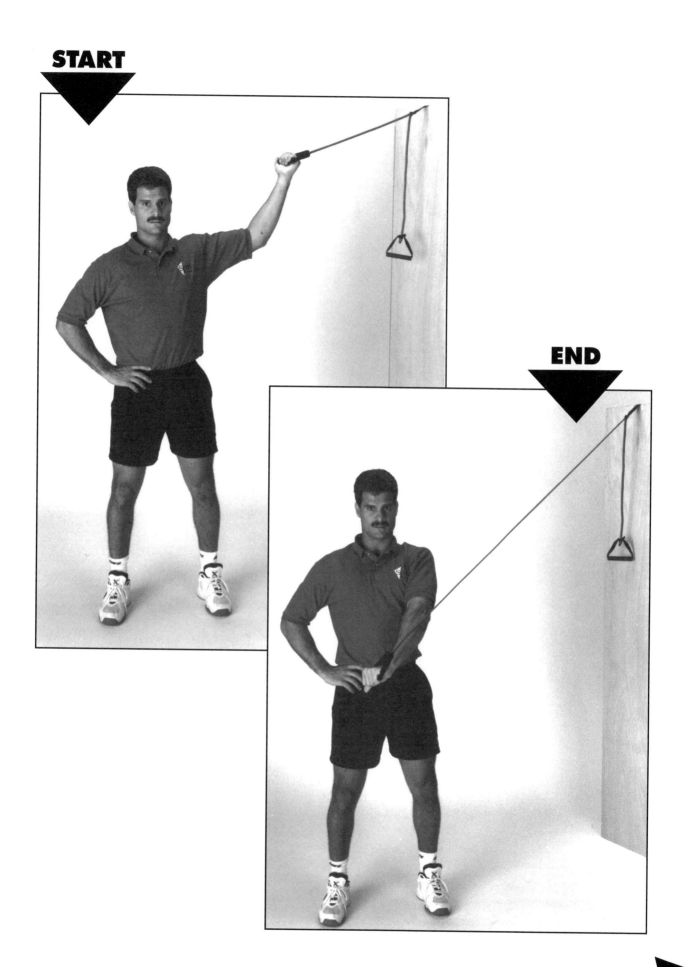

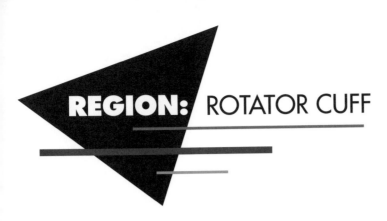

XERTUBE SUPRASPINATUS MOTOR PATTERN
(Supraspinatus)

A. Stand in a square or staggered stance. Place tubing under arch of front foot or both feet and soft knees. Keep hips back, tilt pelvis slightly anterior and lumbar spine neutral.

B. Grasp handles, maintain a slight bend in elbows, rotate shoulders inward, and point thumbs at outer thighs. The rib cage should be lifted up and shoulder blades resting in their natural position.

C. Lift arms upward and away from sides of body. The little finger of each hand should lead arm until 60° of abduction has been performed. This position is more towards shoulder abduction (to the side), but slightly forward of hips.

D. Finish with thumbs pointing down, shoulder blades squeezed together, elbows soft and hands slightly in front of torso.

E. Keep the chest up, rib cage lifted, bellybutton drawn toward spine and the lumbar spine in its neutral curvature.

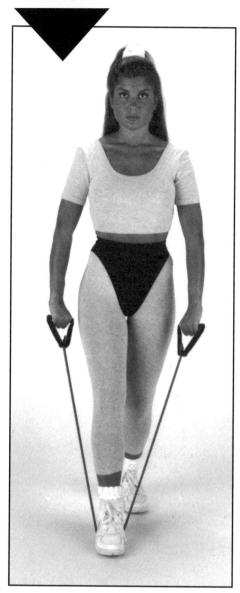

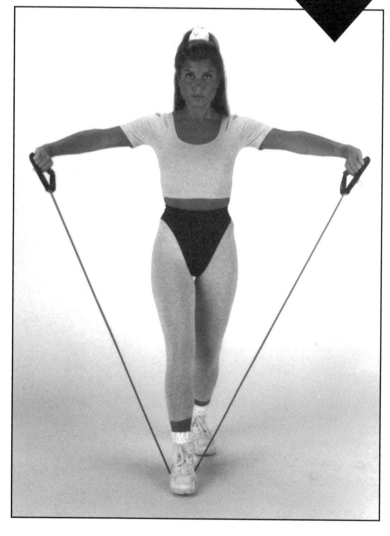

XERTUBE STANDING ARM CURL

(Biceps)

▼ Position of shoulder joint - Neutral

A. Stand in a staggered, narrow or wide stance. Place tubing under arch of front foot or both feet and soften knees. Keep hips back, tilt pelvis slightly anterior and lumbar spine neutral.

B. Grasp handles and straighten arms directly under shoulders with thumbs pointing forward.

C. Bend elbows and gradually turn forearms so palms face ceiling at hip level.

D. Continue bending elbows until fists face ceiling. Palms of hands end facing front portion of shoulders with thumbs pointing out and away from sides of body. Finish with elbows directly under shoulders.

E. Keep the chest up, rib cage lifted, bellybutton drawn toward spine and the lumbar spine in its neutral curvature.

F. This exercise may be performed with one arm at a time by standing on one end of tubing.

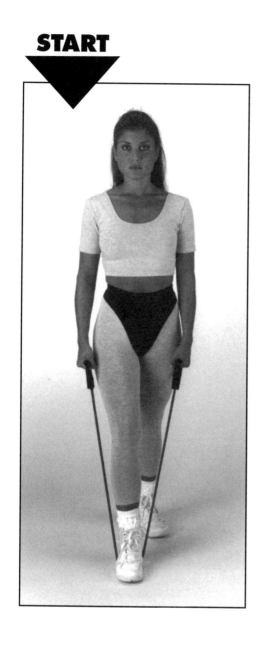

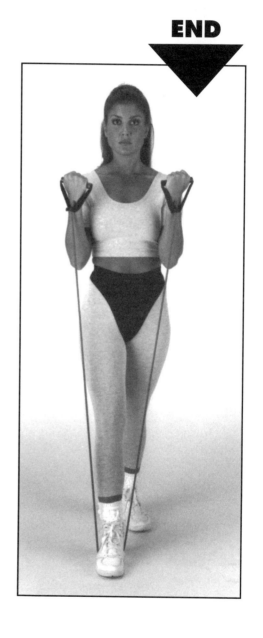

XERTUBE STANDING PREACHER ARM CURL
(Biceps)

▼ Position of shoulder joint - Frontal

A. Anchor tubing at shoulder height, grasp handles and back away from insertion until arms fully lengthen straight out from shoulders.

B. Assume a square stance slightly wider than shoulder width and soften knees. Keep hips back, tilt pelvis slightly anterior and lumbar spine neutral.

C. Keep arms at shoulder height with thumbs facing up.

D. Bend elbows and gradually turn forearms so palms face ceiling. Curl fully ending with palms facing front part of shoulders. Finish with elbows aligned with shoulders.

E. Keep the chest up, rib cage lifted, bellybutton drawn toward spine and the lumbar spine in its neutral curvature.

F. This exercise may be performed with one arm at a time.

THE COMPLETE GUIDE TO **RUBBERIZED RESISTANCE EXERCISES** 129

XERTUBE PARTNER STANDING PREACHER ARM CURL

(Biceps)

▼ Position of shoulder joint - Frontal

A. Exerciser and partner face each other. Two Xertubes are used simultaneously for this exercise. Each person grasps one handle of the same Xertube with the right hand and one handle of the other Xertube with the left.

B. Move away from each other taking steps backward to a desired tension level and assume a staggered lunge stance. Keep knees bent slightly, hips back, pelvis tilted slightly anterior, lumbar spine neutral and lean torso forward slightly. Extend arms fully at shoulder height. The forearms may be positioned with palms facing inward (neutral) or facing upward (supinated).

C. With firm wrists, bend elbows and perform the curling motion while keeping the elbows and upper and lower arms stationary. Keep the forearms in a neutral or supinated position throughout the motion or transition from a neutral to supinated position. Keep the chest expanded, rib cage lifted and bellybutton drawn toward spine.

D. Finish with the elbows directly parallel to the shoulders and knuckles facing the ceiling. The staggered lunge stance must be maintained.

E. Slowly return to the starting position.

**This exercise may be performed with one arm only or in an alternating arm fashion.

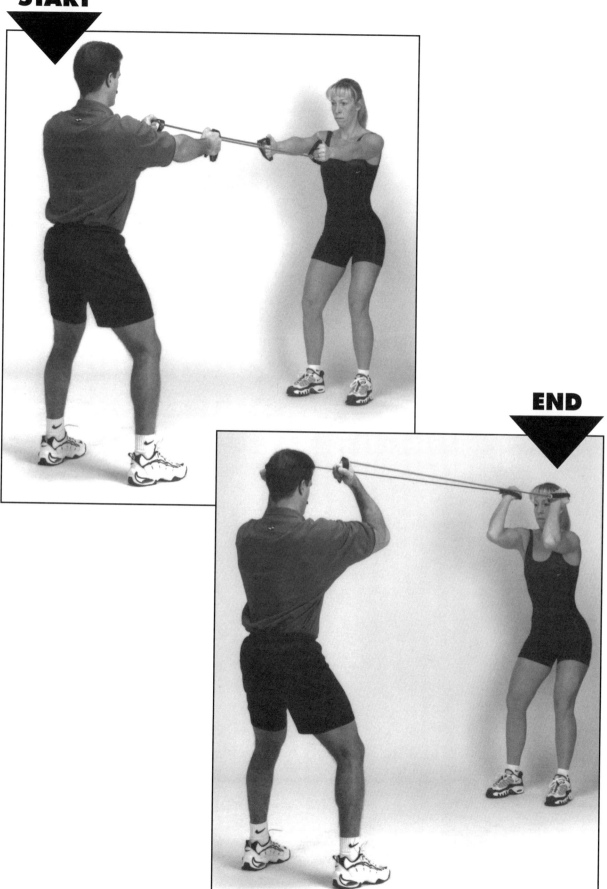

START

END

XERTUBE SEATED PREACHER ARM CURL

(Biceps)

▼ Position of shoulder joint - Frontal

A. Sit with knees comfortably bent, center tubing under middle of both feet. Grasp tubing in between both feet and pull toward you to create a loop. Place loop back over feet.

B. Grasp handles with thumbs up and sit upright. Keep feet together for less resistance and apart for more resistance.

C. OPTION 1 - Bend and flare elbows, turn palms toward chest while curling fully. End with palms of hands in contact with lower chest and knuckles facing each other.

OPTION 2 - Bend elbows and gradually turn forearms so palms face ceiling. Flex shoulders slightly and curl fully, ending with palms facing front of shoulders. Shoulders end flexed approximately 80° with elbows slightly under shoulders.

D. Keep the chest up, rib cage lifted, bellybutton drawn toward spine and the lumbar spine in its neutral curvature.

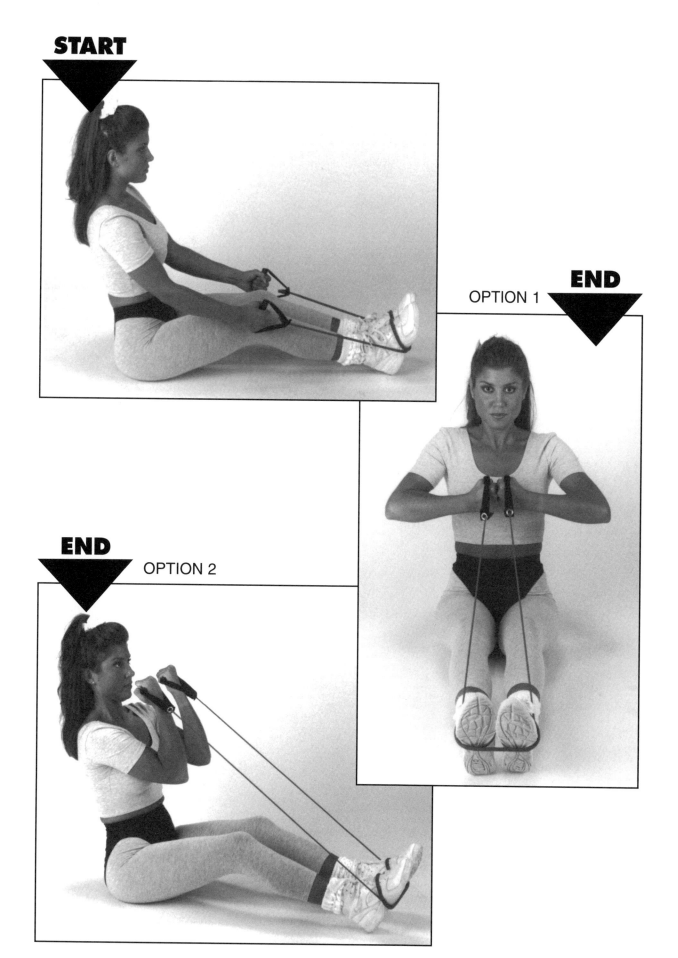

START

END

OPTION 1

END

OPTION 2

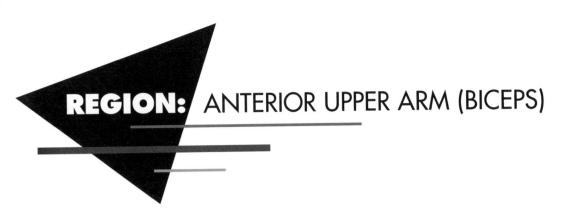

REGION: ANTERIOR UPPER ARM (BICEPS)

XERTUBE BENCH SUPINE PREACHER ARM CURL

(Biceps)

▼ Position of shoulder joint - Frontal

A. Anchor tubing at top of door directly in line with middle of bench. Move bench away from attachment site to place desired tension on tubing once in the starting position. Lie supine with head at end of bench toward attachment site. Place feet on bench with knees bent and raise hands directly over shoulders.

B. Have partner place a handle in each hand (two arms) or handle(s) in one hand (single). Keep the upper arm(s) aligned over shoulder(s) and position forearm(s) with palm(s) facing inward (neutral) or backward (supinated).

**If using one arm, align the insertion with the shoulder of the exercising arm.

C. With firm wrist(s), bend elbow(s) and perform the curling motion while keeping the elbow(s) and upper and lower arm(s) stationary. Keep the forearm(s) in a neutral or supinated position throughout the motion or transition from a neutral to supinated position. Keep the chest expanded, rib cage lifted and bellybutton drawn toward spine.

D. Finish with the elbow(s) directly over the shoulder(s) and knuckles facing behind body.

E. Slowly return to the starting position. If using one arm, align the insertion with the other arm and repeat an equal amount of repetitions.

START

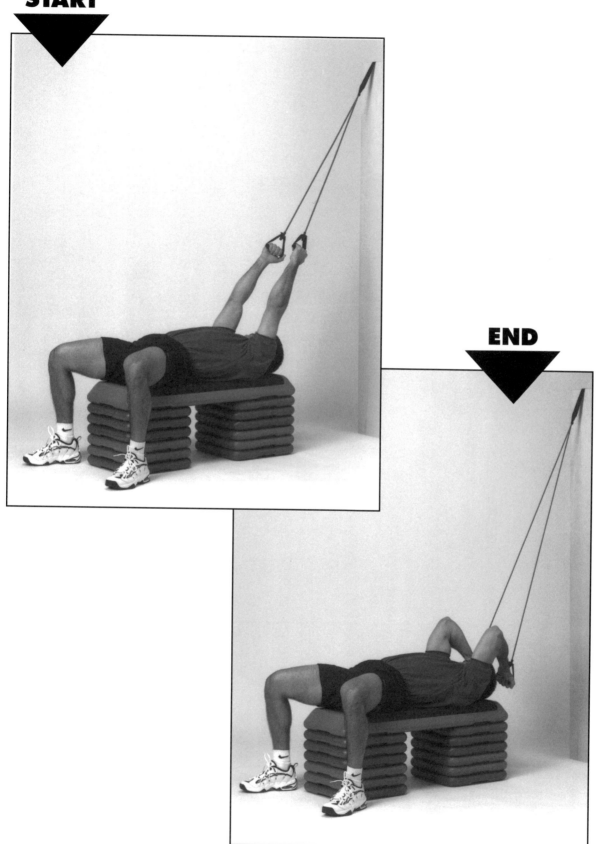

END

REGION: ANTERIOR UPPER ARM (BICEPS)

XERTUBE STANDING ARM CURL
(Biceps)

▼ **Position of shoulder joint - Posterior**

A. Anchor tubing at ankle height. Face away from insertion in a staggered lunge position. Soften knees, keep hips back, tilt pelvis slightly anterior and lumbar spine neutral.

B. Grasp handles and position arms behind body in a thumbs forward position.

C. Keeping elbows behind torso, bend at elbow and gradually turn forearms so palms face ceiling. Curl fully, ending with hands parallel to outer-lower portion of chest.

D. Keep the chest up, rib cage lifted, bellybutton drawn toward spine and the lumbar spine in its neutral curvature.

TECH TIPS

This exercise may be performed one side at a time.

START

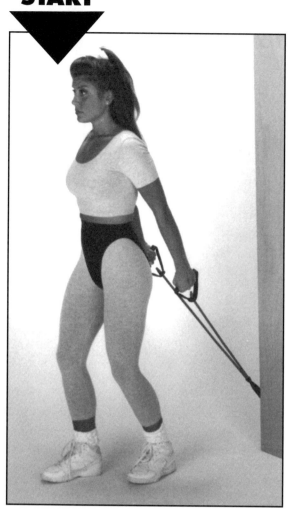

END

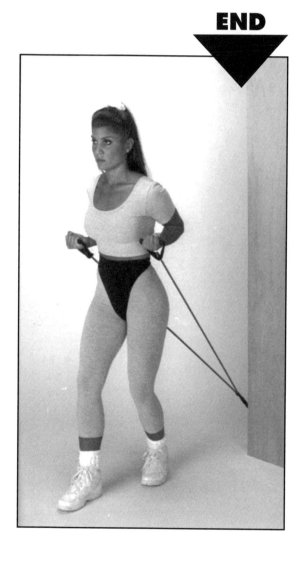

STEP XERTUBE STANDING ARM CURL
(Biceps)

▼ Position of shoulder joint - Neutral

A. Tubing is secured through step strap at outside attachment.

B. Grasp tubing and stand on step nearest to step strap.

C. Face attachment and stand in a square stance. Soften knees, keep hips back, tilt pelvis slightly anterior and lumbar spine neutral.

D. Straighten arms directly under shoulders with thumbs pointing forward.

E. Bend elbows and gradually turn forearms so palms face ceiling at hip level.

F. Continue bending elbows until fists face ceiling. Palms of hands end facing front portion of shoulders with thumbs pointing out and away from sides of body. Finish with elbows directly under shoulders.

G. Keep the chest up, rib cage lifted, bellybutton drawn toward spine and the lumbar spine in its neutral curvature.

TECH TIPS
   This exercise may be performed one side at a time.

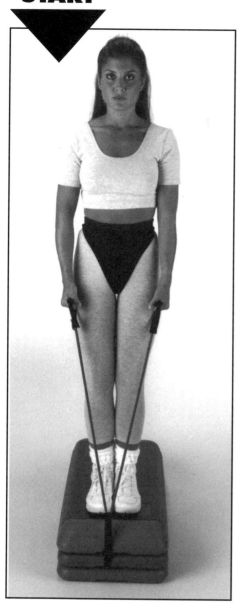

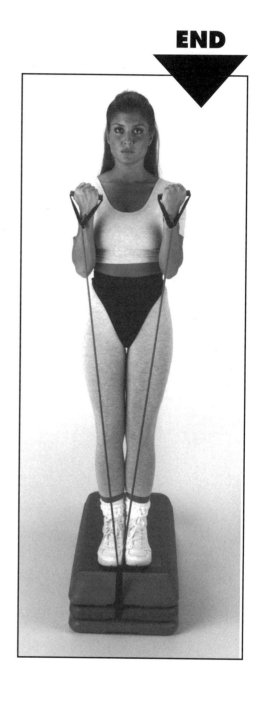

STEP XERTUBE STANDING PREACHER ARM CURL

(Biceps)

▼ Position of shoulder joint - Frontal

A. Tubing is secured through step strap at outside attachment.

B. Grasp handles and stand on step farthest from step strap.

C. Face attachment and stand in a narrow, staggered lunge stance. Soften knees, keep hips back, tilt pelvis slightly anterior and lumbar spine neutral.

D. Flex shoulders 45° and straighten arms in alignment with shoulders with palms of hands facing up.

E. Bend elbows and curl fully ending with the palms facing front part of shoulders. Finish with shoulders flexed 45°.

F. Keep the chest up, rib cage lifted, bellybutton drawn toward spine and the lumbar spine in its neutral curvature.

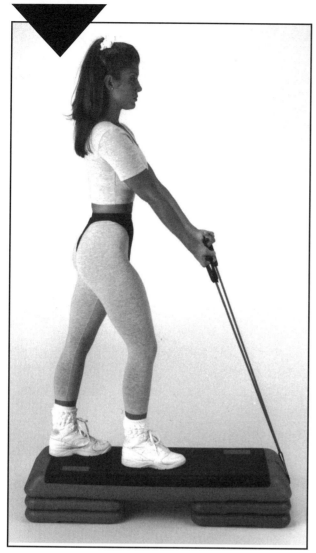

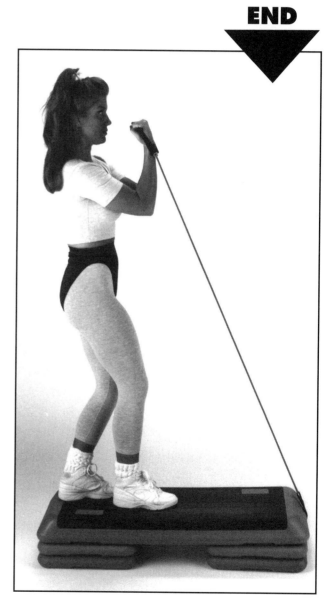

STEP XERTUBE STANDING ARM CURL
(Biceps)

▼ **Position of shoulder joint - Posterior**

A. Tubing is secured through step strap at outside attachment. Grasp handles and stand on step farthest from step strap.

B. Face away from attachment site so that tubing pulls from behind body. Keep one foot directly over middle of step block and place the other foot on floor, creating a staggered lunge stance. Soften knees, keep hips back, tilt pelvis slightly anterior and lumbar spine neutral.

C. Position arms behind body in a thumbs forward position.

D. Keeping elbows behind torso, bend elbows and progressively turn forearms so palms face ceiling.

E. Keep the chest up, rib cage lifted, bellybutton drawn toward spine and the lumbar spine in its neutral curvature.

TECH TIPS

If end of step at attachment site rises up during the curling motion, move foot on step toward attachment site.

START

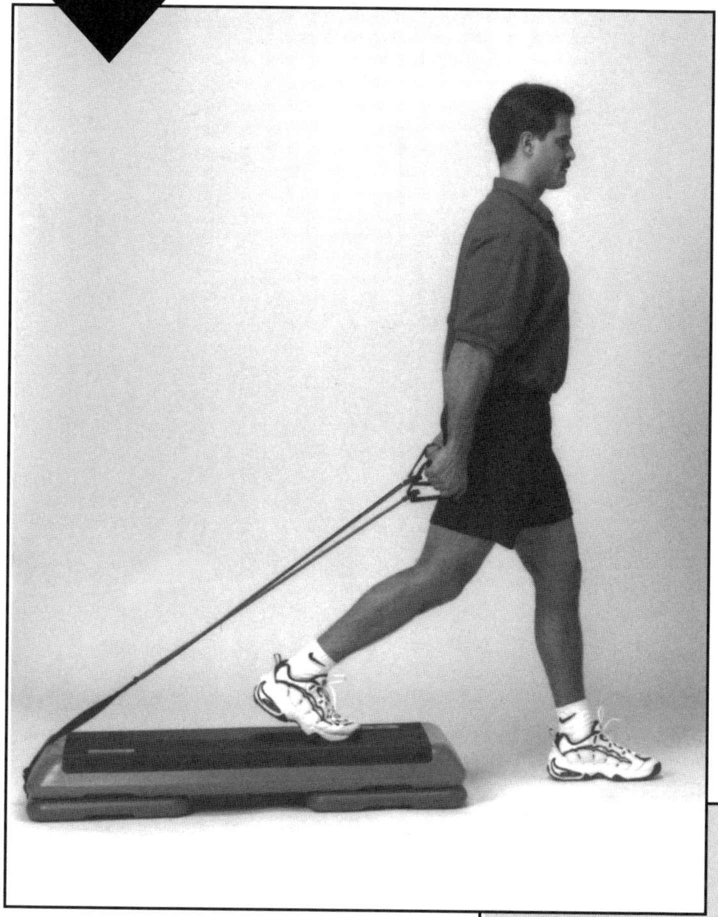

END

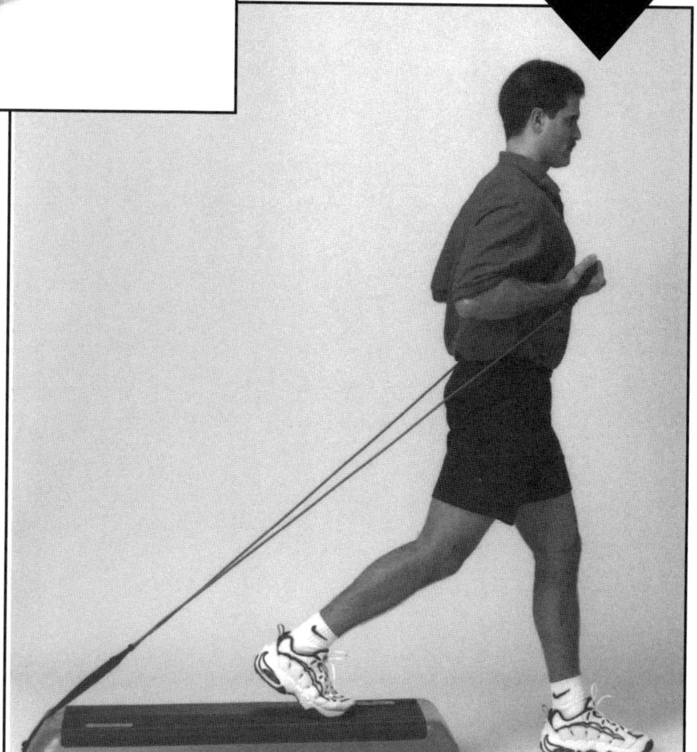

XERTUBE STANDING PRESS DOWN

(Triceps)

▼ Position of shoulder joint - Neutral

A. Anchor tubing above head height and assume a square stance slightly wider than shoulder width and soften knees. Kneel in a staggered lunge position if more resistance is needed. Lean upper torso forward slightly, keep hips back, tilt pelvis slightly anterior and lumbar spine neutral.

B. Grasp handles, bend elbows and keep them directly under shoulders.

C. Hands begin slightly higher than elbows with palms facing each other and thumbs pointing upward.

D. With firm wrists, press down and gradually turn forearms downward, straightening arms fully. End with palms facing thighs, knuckles facing floor and elbows directly under shoulders.

E. Keep the chest up, rib cage lifted, bellybutton drawn toward spine and the lumbar spine in its neutral curvature.

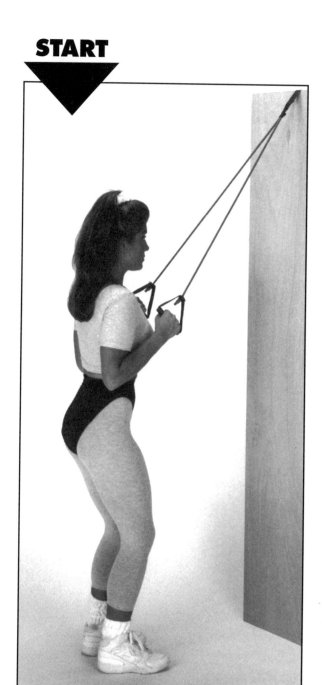

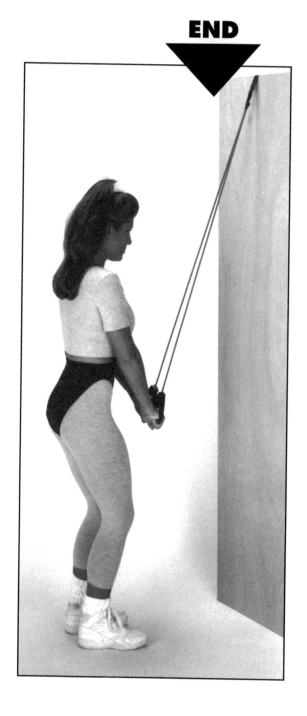

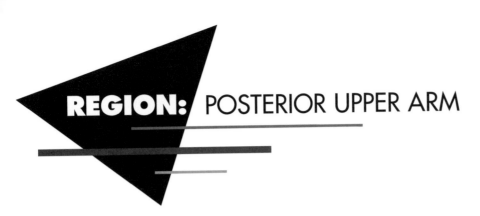

XERTUBE STANDING SINGLE ARM SUPINATED GRIP PRESS DOWN

(Triceps)

▼ Position of shoulder joint - Neutral

A. Anchor tubing at top of door when standing. Face tubing with shoulder of exercising arm aligned with attachment site.

B. Grasp handle(s) in hand aligned with insertion and move away from attachment site to desired tension level and assume a quarter-squat position. Keep hips back, pelvis tilted slightly anterior, lumbar spine neutral and torso slightly forward (athletic position). Bend elbow and position it directly under shoulder with palm facing up (supinated). The upper and lower arm angle should be 90°.

C. With a firm wrist, press down and back while keeping upper arm and elbow stationary. Keep the forearm in a supinated position throughout the motion. Keep the chest expanded, rib cage lifted and bellybutton drawn toward spine.

D. Finish with hand behind hip, elbow fully extended and palm facing forward (supinated). The quarter-squat athletic position must be maintained.

E. Slowly return to the starting position. Align the insertion with the other arm and repeat an equal amount of repetitions.

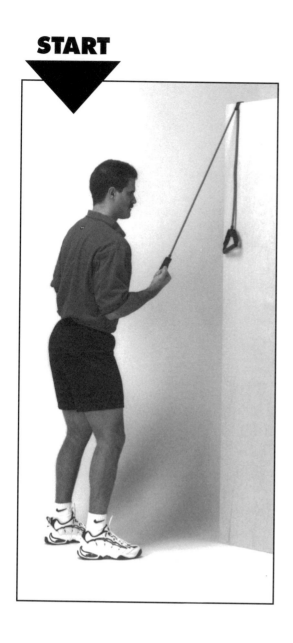

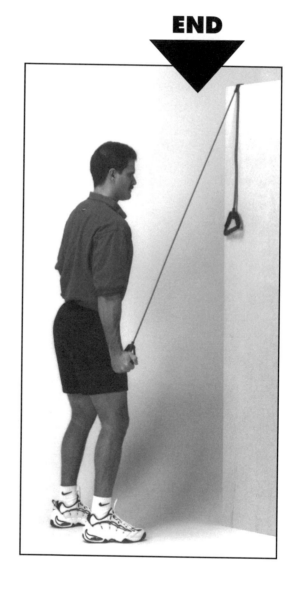

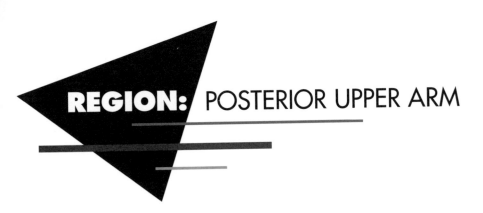

REGION: POSTERIOR UPPER ARM

XERTUBE STANDING OVERHEAD PRESS UP
(Triceps)

▼ **Position of shoulder joint - Frontal**

A. Stand in a narrow, staggered lunge stance. Place tubing under arch of rear foot and soften both knees. Keep hips back, tilt pelvis slightly anterior and lumbar spine neutral.

B. Grasp handles and raise elbows directly over shoulders with palms facing each other and thumbs pointing down.

C. With firm wrists, press up and gradually pronate forearms, straightening arms fully. End with hands directly over shoulders and palms facing forward with knuckles facing ceiling.

D. Keep the chest up, rib cage lifted, bellybutton drawn toward spine and the lumbar spine in its neutral curvature.

> **TECH TIPS**
> This exercise may be performed one arm at a time by standing on one end of tubing. If the exerciser is unable to stabilize the spine while using two arms, one arm should be used.

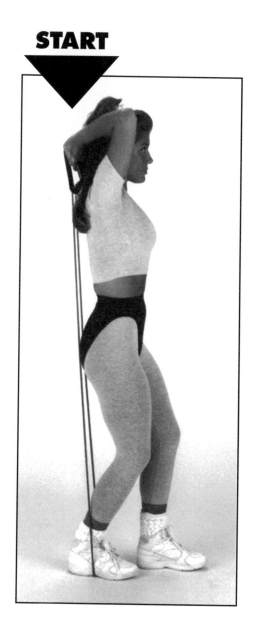

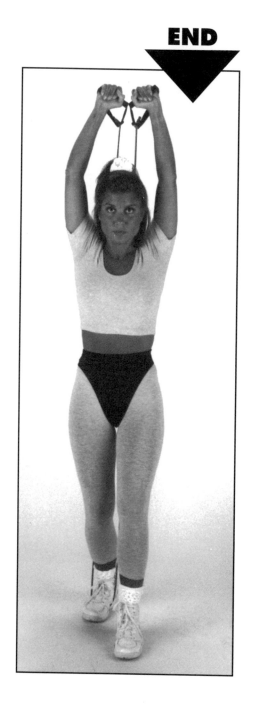

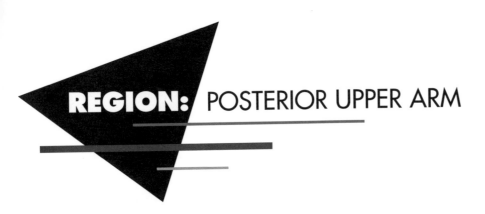

XERTUBE BENCH SUPINE PRESS UP
(Triceps)

▼ Position of shoulder joint - Frontal

A. Anchor tubing at ankle height directly in line with middle of bench. Move bench away from attachment site to place desired tension on tubing once in the starting position. Lie supine with head at end of bench toward attachment site. Place feet on bench with knees bent and raise hands directly over shoulders with palms facing each other.

**If using one arm, align the insertion with the shoulder of the exercising arm.

B. Have partner place a handle in each hand (two arms) or handle(s) in one hand (single arm). Bend elbow(s) and position directly over shoulder(s) with hand(s) positioned just above top of ear(s). The forearm(s) may be positioned with palm(s) facing up (pronated), facing inward (neutral) or facing back (supinated).

C. With firm wrist(s), press upward while keeping elbow(s) and upper and lower arm(s) stationary. Keep the forearm(s) in a pronated, neutral or supinated position throughout the motion or transition from a neutral to pronated position. Keep the chest expanded, rib cage lifted and bellybutton drawn toward spine.

D. Finish with the hand(s) directly over the shoulder(s) with knuckles facing the ceiling.

E. Slowly return to the starting position. If using one arm, align the insertion with the other arm and repeat an equal amount of repetitions.

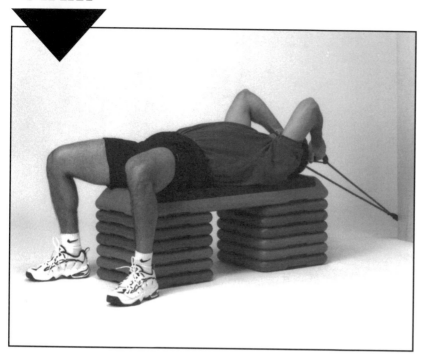

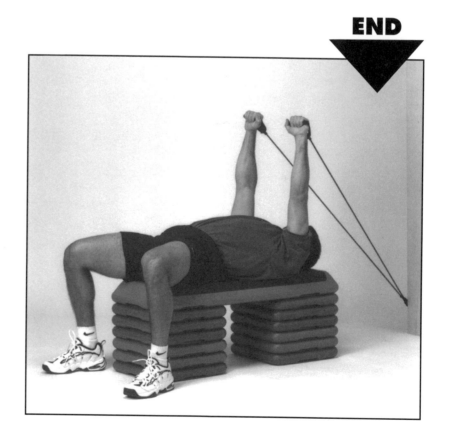

XERTUBE STANDING OVERHEAD PRESS OUT

(Triceps)

▼ Position of shoulder joint - Frontal

A. Anchor tubing above head height. Grasp handles and face away from tubing insertion so it pulls from behind.

B. Stand in a narrow, staggered lunge stance and soften both knees. Keep hips back, tilt pelvis slightly anterior and lumbar spine neutral.

C. Bend arms and position elbows directly in front of shoulders with upper arms parallel to floor. Position palms of hands along side of ears.

D. Lean slightly forward with upper torso. With firm wrists, press out and gradually turn forearms while straightening arms fully. End with palms facing down and hands in direct line with shoulders.

E. Keep the chest up, rib cage lifted, bellybutton drawn toward spine and the lumbar spine in its neutral curvature.

TECH TIPS
This exercise may be performed one arm at a time. If the exerciser is unable to stabilize the spine when using two arms, one arm should be used.

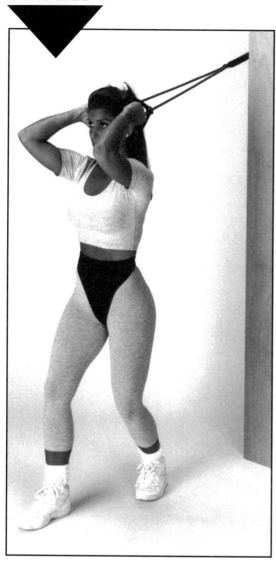

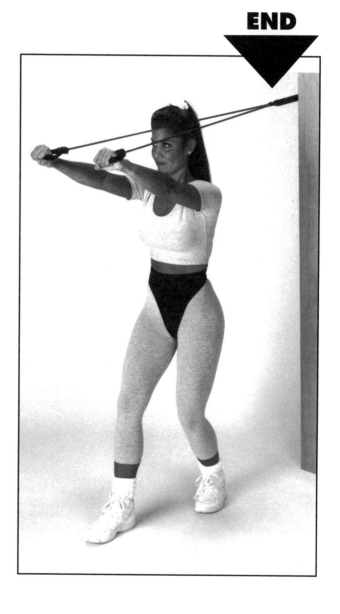

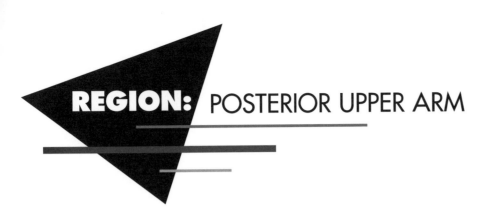

REGION: POSTERIOR UPPER ARM

XERTUBE STANDING PRESS BACK
(Triceps)

▼ Position of shoulder joint - Posterior

A. Anchor tubing at waist height, grasp handles with thumbs pointing up.

B. Face attachment in a narrow staggered lunge position and soften knees. Keep hips back, tilt pelvis slightly anterior and lumbar spine neutral.

C. Bend elbows forming two right angles and position them behind torso so shoulder blades are squeezed together.

D. Start with hands parallel to outer-lower portion of chest in a thumbs up position. With firm wrists, press down and back and gradually turn forearms back while straightening arms fully. End with palms facing back and elbows behind torso.

E. Keep the chest up, rib cage lifted, bellybutton drawn toward spine and the lumbar spine in its neutral curvature.

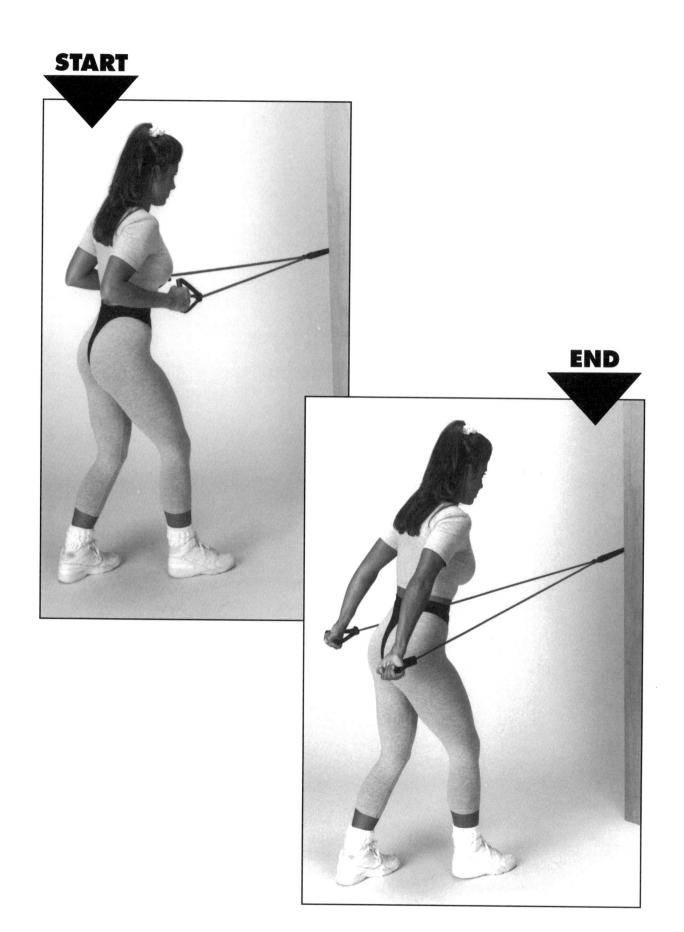

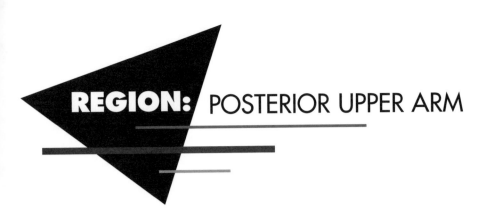

REGION: POSTERIOR UPPER ARM

XERTUBE PARTNER STANDING PRESS BACK
(Triceps)

▼ Position of shoulder joint - Posterior

A. Exerciser and partner stand facing each other. Two Xertubes are used simultaneously for this exercise. Each person grasps one handle of the same Xertube with the right hand and one handle of the other Xertube with the left.

B. Move away from each other taking steps backward to a desired tension level and assume a staggered lunge stance. Keep knees bent slightly, hips back, pelvis tilted slightly anterior, lumbar spine neutral and lean torso forward slightly. Bend elbows and position behind torso with shoulder blades squeezed toward spine and palms facing down (pronated), facing inward (neutral), facing up (supinated). The upper and lower arm angle should be 90°.

C. With firm wrists, press back while keeping upper arms and elbows stationary. Keep the forearms in a pronated, neutral or supinated position throughout the motion or transition from a neutral to pronated position. Keep the chest expanded, rib cage lifted, and bellybutton drawn toward spine.

D. Finish with hands behind hips, elbows fully extended and palms facing backward (pronated), toward each other (neutral), or forward (supinated). The staggered lunge stance must be maintained.

E. Slowly return to the starting position.

TECH TIPS
This exercise may be performed one arm at a time or in an alternating arm fashion. If the exerciser is unable to stabilize the spine with two arms, one arm should be used.

START

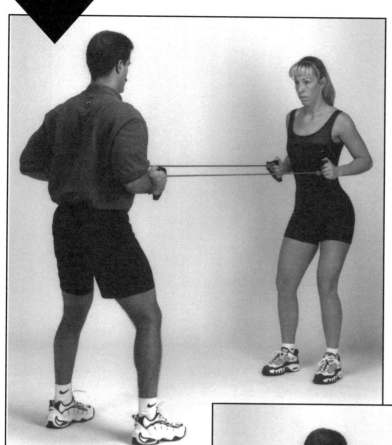

END

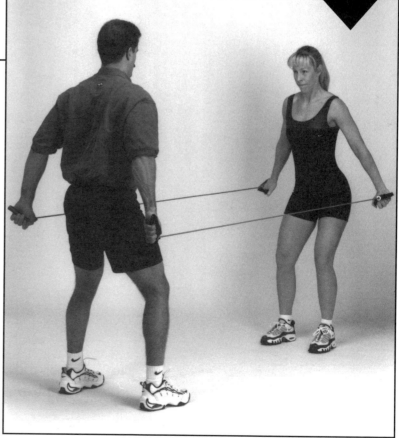

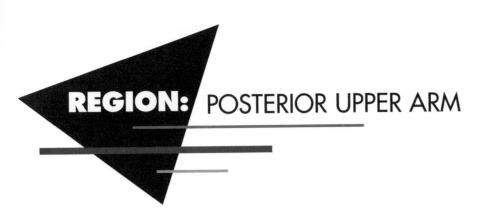

REGION: POSTERIOR UPPER ARM

STEP XERTUBE   STANDING OVERHEAD PRESS UP

(Triceps)

▼   **Position of shoulder joint - Frontal**

A. Tubing is secured through step strap at outside attachment.

B. Grasp handles and stand on step nearest to step strap.

C. Face away from attachment in a narrow, staggered lunge position and soften both knees. Keep hips back, tilt pelvis slightly anterior and lumbar spine neutral.

D. Raise elbows directly over shoulders with palms facing each other and thumbs pointing down.

E. With firm wrists, press up and gradually turn forearms, straightening arms fully. End with hands directly over shoulders and palms facing forward with knuckles facing ceiling.

F. Keep the chest up, rib cage lifted, bellybutton drawn toward spine and the lumbar spine in its neutral curvature.

G. Turn the opposite direction and repeat equal amounts of repetitions with other hand.

> ### TECH TIPS
> This exercise may be performed one arm at a time. If the exerciser is unable to stabilize the spine with two arms, one arm should be used.

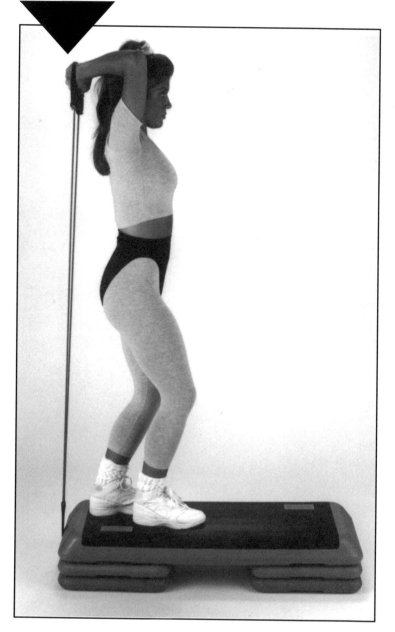

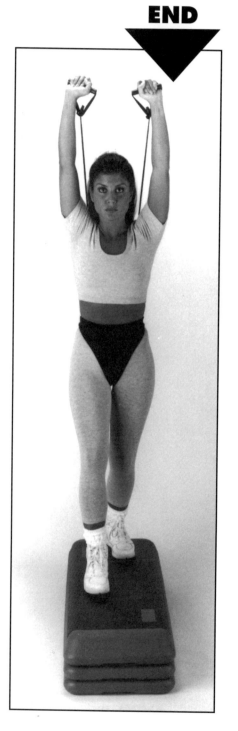

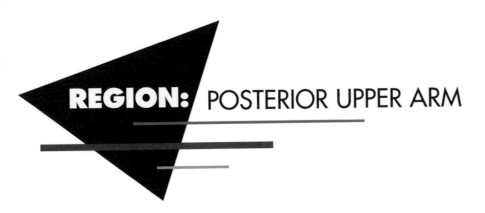

STEP XERTUBE STANDING PRESS BACK

(Triceps)

▼ **Position of shoulder joint - Posterior**

A. Tubing is secured through step strap at outside attachment. Grasp handles and stand on step farthest from step strap facing attachment site.

B. Keep one foot directly over middle of step block and place other foot on floor behind body, creating a staggered lunge stance. Assume a quarter-squat position, keep hips back, tilt pelvis slightly anterior and lumbar spine neutral.

C. Bend elbows forming two right angles and position them behind torso so shoulder blades are squeezed together.

D. Start with hands parallel to outer - lower portion of chest in a thumbs up position. With firm wrists, press down and back and gradually turn forearms back while straightening arms fully. End with palms facing back and elbows behind torso.

E. Keep the chest up, rib cage lifted, bellybutton drawn toward spine and the lumbar spine in its neutral curvature.

> **TECH TIPS**
> **If end of step at attachment site rises up during the press back motion, move foot on step toward attachment site.**

START

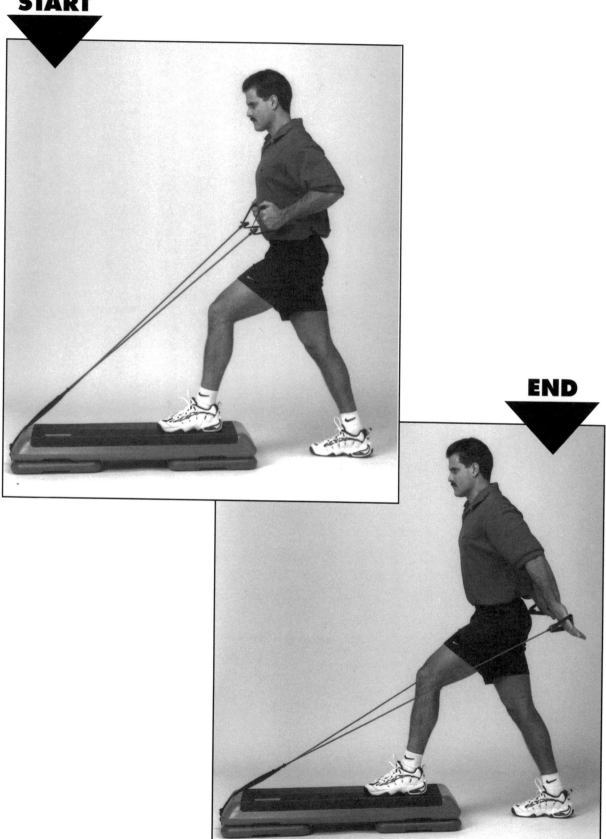

END

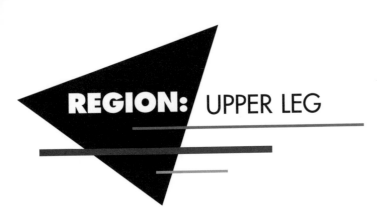

REGION: UPPER LEG

XERTUBE BACK SQUAT
(Quadriceps/Hamstrings/Gluteals)

A. Position feet in a moderate stance with big toes directly under hips and toes out slightly (20° - 30° of external hip rotation).

B. Place tubing under arches of both feet. Grasp handles and raise hands to shoulder height.

C. Keep head over hips and focus eyes slightly higher than head. Keep chest expanded, rib cage lifted, shoulder blades squeezed together and bellybutton drawn toward spine.

D. Bend knees, tilt pelvis forward (hips back) and maintain natural arch in low back. Sit back until upper legs are just above parallel in relation to floor. The lower back must maintain a neutral curvature, stop the descent when lower back loses its curvature (flexes), even if a parallel position is not achieved.

E. Keep heels down with body weight over ankles and knees over mid-foot. Middle of kneecapss align with last two toes at bottom of squat.

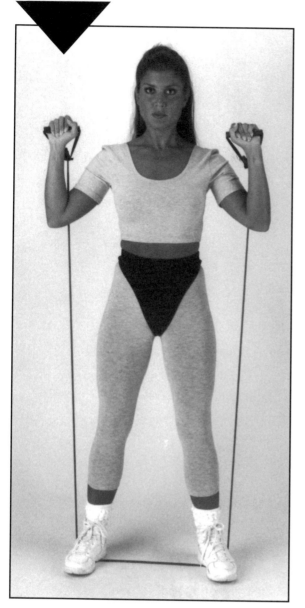

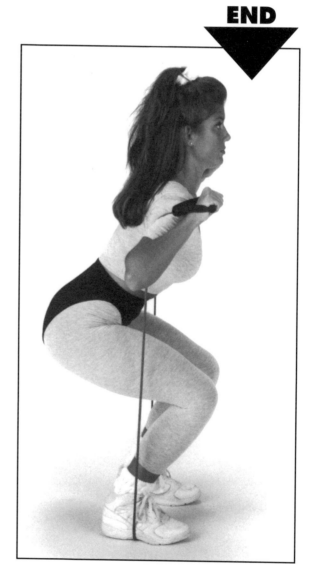

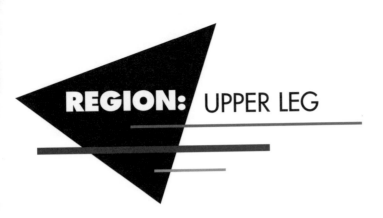

XERTUBE BENT TRAIL LEG LUNGE
(Quadriceps/Hamstrings/Gluteals)

A. Stand in a narrow staggered lunge stance and place tubing under arch of front foot.

B. Grasp handles and raise hands to shoulder height.

C. Take a drop step with other leg and land on ball of foot. Bend knees and descend to form a 90° angle with upper and lower portion of each leg. The kneecap of lead leg should be approximately over the mid-foot. Keep heel down and weight distributed evenly through front foot. Heel of trail leg is up off floor, knee slightly behind hips and ball of foot is in contact with floor.

D. Keep head over hips and eyes focused directly forward. Keep chest expanded, rib cage lifted, shoulder blades squeezed together, bellybutton drawn toward spine and the lumbar spine in its neutral curvature.

E. STATIONARY - Keep feet in this position, straighten both lead and trail legs simultaneously. Stand tall through ball of trail leg foot and squeeze gluteal muscles. **DYNAMIC -** Return to start position, (point A) and repeat drop step (point C).

F. Place tubing under arch of other foot and repeat equal amounts of repetitions with other leg.

START/END

DYNAMIC

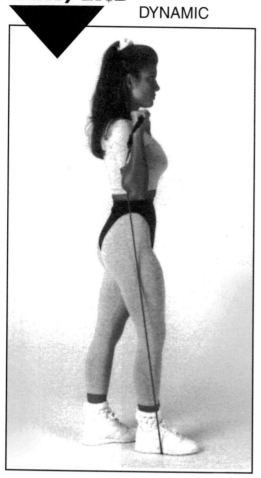

STATIONARY **START/END**

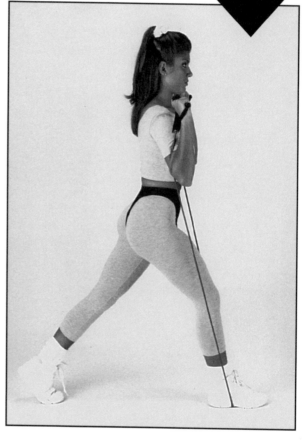

MID

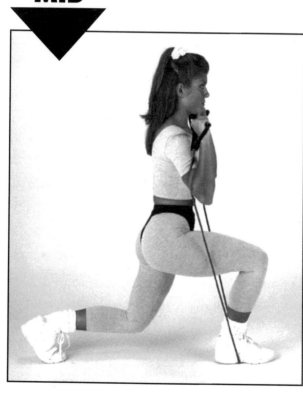

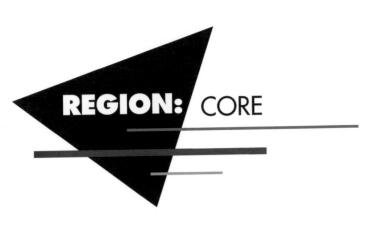

XERTUBE STANDING TORSO ROTATION
(Internal and External Obliques, Posterior Spinal Rotators)

A. Anchor tubing between bellybutton and lower sternum when standing. Position torso parallel to and behind attachment site approximately 12".

B. Grasp handle(s) with hand furthest from attachment site and place other hand over it. Move away from attachment site to desired tension level and assume a quarter-squat position. Keep hips back, pelvis tilted slightly anterior, lumber spine neutral, and lean torso forward slightly (athletic position). Extend arms straight out from lower chest and keep arm furthest from attachment site straightened throughout.

C. When rotating to the left, start by rotating torso to the right approximately one-quarter turn (45°) with eyes focused forward. Keep arms extended, rib cage lifted and bellybutton drawn toward spine while rotating torso to the left. It is extremely important not to pull the tubing with the arms, but to rotate using only the core musculature. The arms should act as an extension of the torso.

D. End with the eyes focused forward and torso fully rotated to the left or one-quarter turn (45°) from center. The quarter-squat athletic position must be maintained throughout.

E. Slowly rotate back to the starting position. Turn the opposite direction and repeat an equal amount of repetitions.

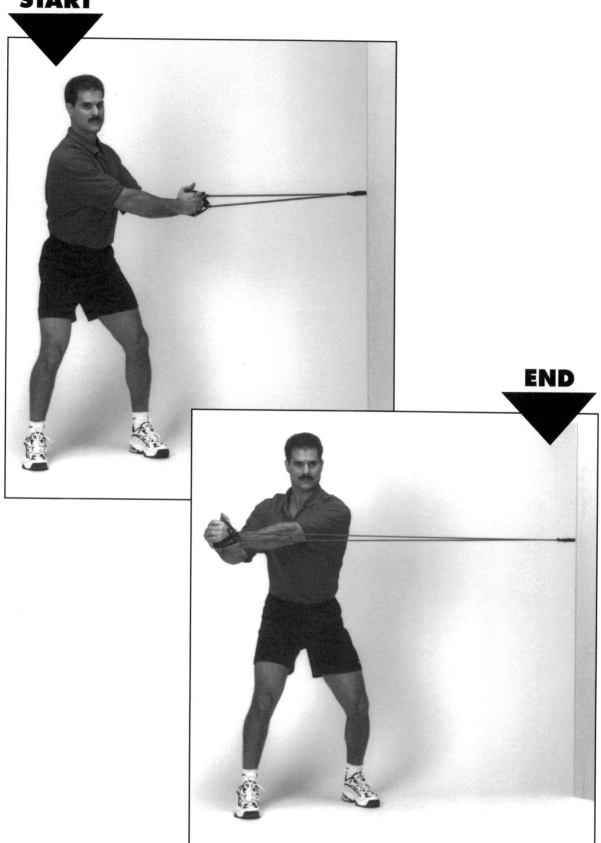

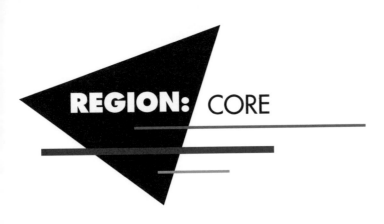

XERTUBE PARTNER STANDING TORSO ROTATION

(Internal And External Obliques, Posterior Spinal Rotators)

A. Exerciser stands across from partner approximately two feet and they align right shoulders. Each person grasps one handle with the left hand and places his/her right hand over it.

**For greater tension use 2 Xertubes.

B. Move away from each other taking steps laterally to a desired tension level and assume a quarter-squat position. Keep hips back, pelvis tilted slightly anterior, lumbar spine neutral and lean torso forward slightly (athletic position). Extend arms straight out from lower chest and keep left arm straightened throughout.

C. When rotating to the left, start by rotating torso to the right approximately one-quarter turn (45°) with eyes focused forward. Keep arms extended, rib cage lifted and bellybutton drawn toward spine while rotating torso to the left. It is extremely important not to pull the tubing with the arms, but to rotate using only the core musculature. The arms should act as an extension of the torso.

D. End with the eyes focused forward and torso fully rotated to the left or one-quarter turn (45°) from center. The quarter-squat athletic position must be maintained throughout.

E. Slowly rotate back to the starting position. Each partner walks forward two feet, turns and faces the opposite direction and repeats an equal amount of repetitions.

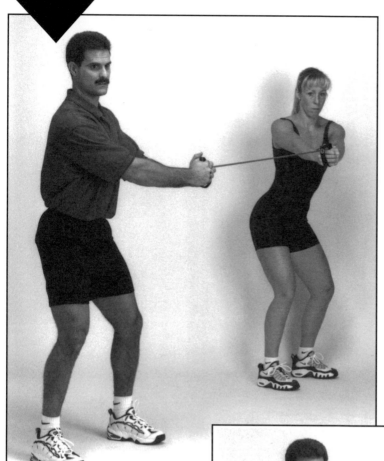

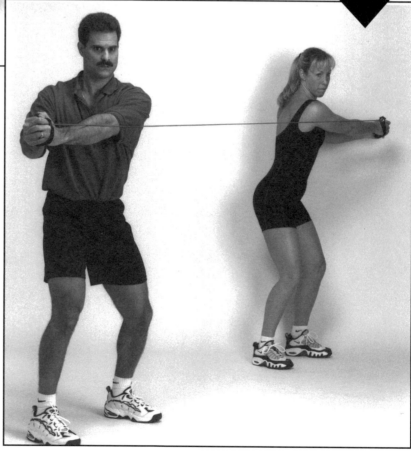

THE COMPLETE GUIDE TO **RUBBERIZED RESISTANCE EXERCISES** **169**

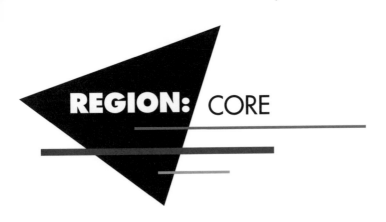

XERTUBE STANDING SIDE BEND

(Internal Obliques, Quadratus Lumborum)

A. Anchor tubing at top of door when standing. Position torso parallel to attachment site.

B. Grasp handle(s) with hand furthest from attachment site and place other hand over it. Move away from attachment site to desired tension level and assume a quarter-squat position. Keep hips back, pelvis tilted slightly anterior, lumbar spine neutral and lean torso forward slightly (athletic position). Extend arms straight over head and keep arm furthest from attachment site straightened throughout.

C. When side bending to the left, start by side bending to the right, placing a pre-stretch on the left side. A gentle stretch should be felt on the left side between the outer hip and lower ribs. While bending to the left, keep the chest up, rib cage expanded, arms as straight as possible and bellybutton drawn toward spine. Focus on the bending motion and the closing of the lower ribs down on the outer hip. The bicep of the right arm should contact the right ear.

D. The arms should be used as an extension of the torso and should not pull excessively. The hips and pelvis should remain stationary with the eyes focused straight ahead. Do not allow the pelvis to shift toward the attachment site upon side bending. The quarter-squat athletic position must be maintained throughout.

E. Slowly side bend back to the starting position. Turn body the opposite direction and repeat an equal amount of repetitions.

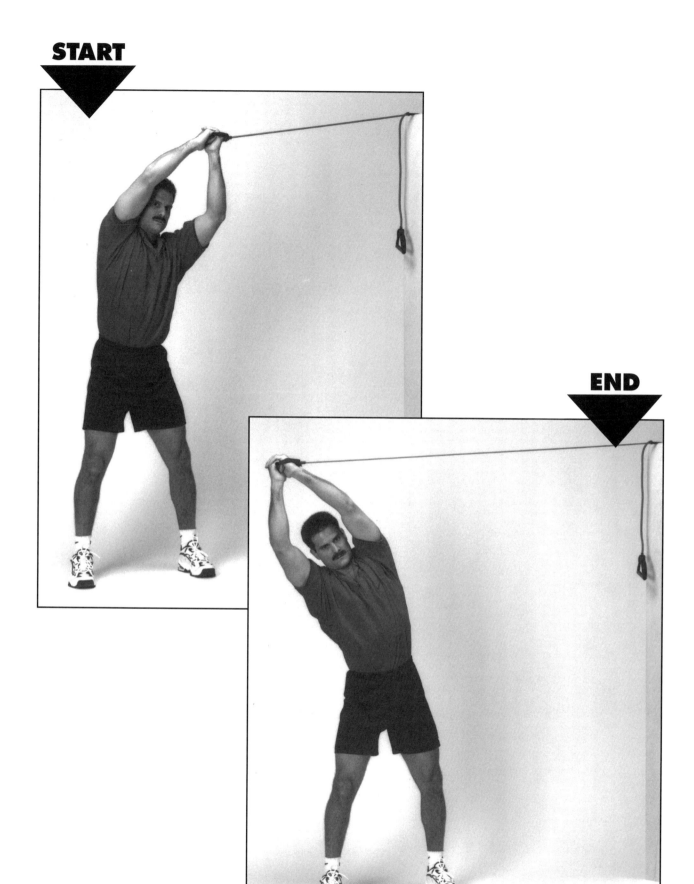

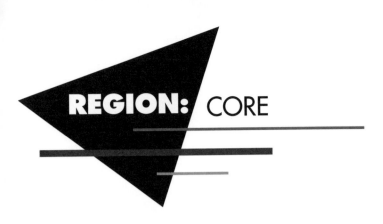

XERTUBE STANDING WOOD CHOP

(Internal And External Obliques, Posterior Spinal Rotators)

A. Anchor tubing at top of door when standing. Position torso parallel to and forward of attachment site approximately 12".

B. Grasp handle(s) with hand furthest from attachment site and place other hand over it. Move away from attachment site to desired tension level and assume lunge stance with the leg furthest away from attachment site forward. Bend knees slightly, keep hips back, tilt pelvis slightly anterior, keep lumbar spine neutral and lean torso forward slightly. Raise arms up and across body toward attachment site. The arm furthest from the attachment site should be kept straight throughout the motion. The chin should be resting against this shoulder in the starting position with the torso rotated one-quarter turn (45°) toward attachment site.

C. The wood chop action should be a diagonal motion biasing spinal rotation with slight flexion. Keep the arms extended, rib cage lifted and bellybutton drawn toward spine while rotating the torso using the downward chopping motion. Internal hip rotation simultaneously occurs from the hip of the back leg when performing the wood chop action.

D. The hands should end slightly outside the mid-thigh with the arms straight and torso rotated one-quarter turn (45°) away from neutral with a slight forward lean. The eyes should focus forward of the foot of the lead leg. The starting lunge stance must be maintained, but the hip of the back leg should naturally rotate inward while the heel lifts slightly. The rib cage should be lifted high, lumbar curvature neutral (not rounded) and bellybutton drawn toward spine.

E. The arms should act as an extension of the torso and should not be used to pull excessively.

F. Slowly reverse the chopping motion to the starting position. Turn body the opposite direction and repeat an equal amount of repetitions.

START

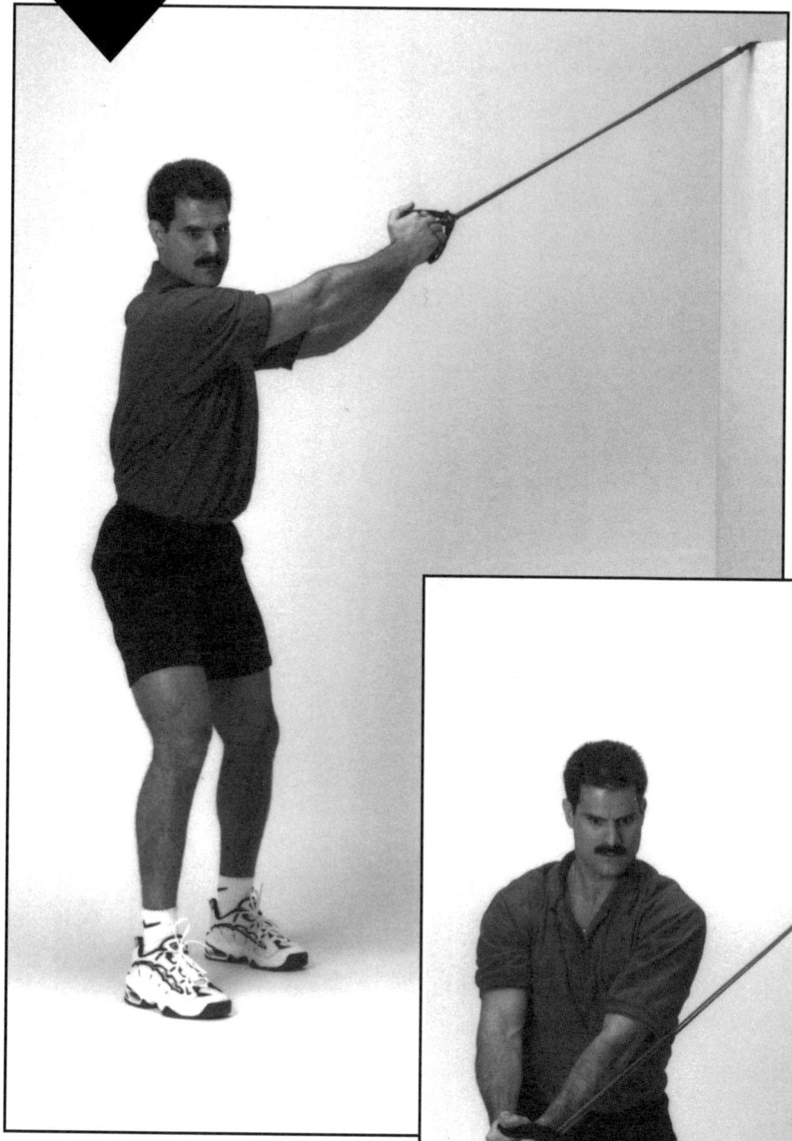

END

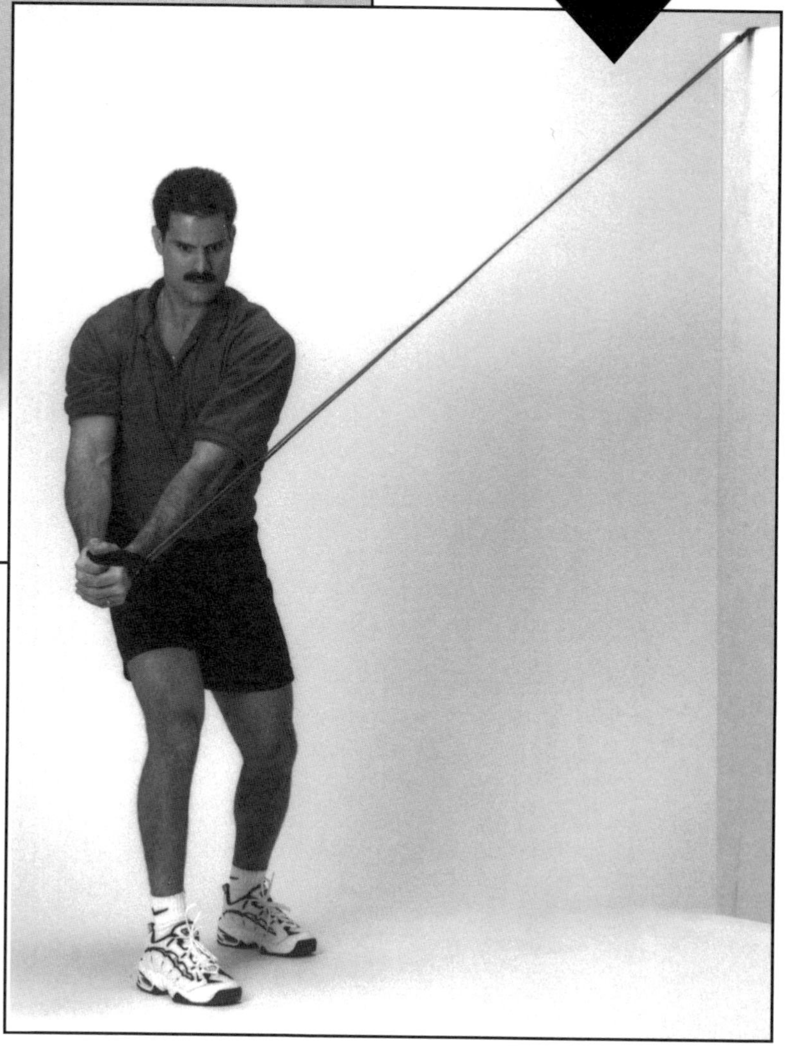

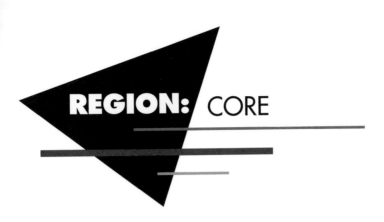

XERTUBE STANDING REVERSE WOOD CHOP
(Internal And External Obliques, Posterior Spinal Rotators)

A. Anchor tubing at ankle height when standing. Position torso parallel to and forward of attachment site approximately 12".

B. Grasp handle(s) with hand furthest from attachment site and place other hand over it. Move away from attachment site to desired tension level and assume a half-squat position. Keep hips back, pelvis tilted slightly anterior, lumbar spine neutral and lean torso forward slightly (athletic position). Straighten arms and rotate torso approximately one-quarter turn toward the attachment site with hands slightly outside mid-thigh.

C. The reverse wood chop (upward arc) action should be a diagonal motion biasing spinal rotation with slight spinal extension. Internal hip rotation simultaneously occurs from the hip closest to the attachment site when rising from the half-squat. Keep the arms extended, rib cage lifted, eyes focused forward and bellybutton drawn toward spine while performing the reverse chopping motion.

D. The hands should end slightly above and lateral to the opposite shoulder with thumbs pointing back. The hip closest to the attachment site should be rotated internally with heel elevated and toes turned inward. The arm closest to the attachment site should be rotated approximately one-quarter turn from neutral. The rib cage should be lifted high, eyes focused forward, lumbar curvature neutral and bellybutton drawn toward spine.

E. The arms should act as an extension of the torso and should not be used to pull excessively.

F. Slowly reverse the chopping motion to the starting position. Turn body the opposite direction and repeat an equal amount of repetitions.

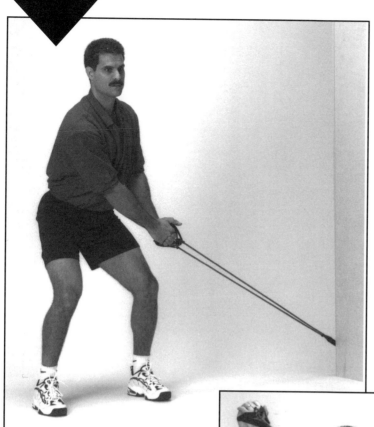

END

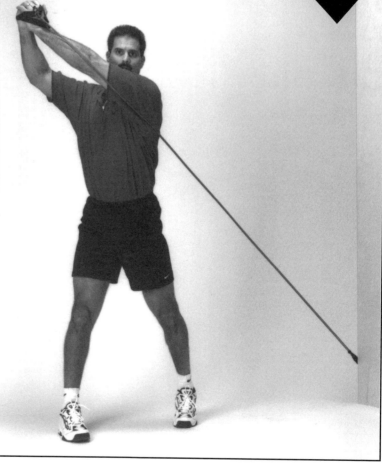

XERCISE BAR

XERCISE BAR™ RESISTANCE CHART

COLOR	RESISTANCE
YELLOW	BEGINNER/INTERMEDIATE
RED	INTERMEDIATE/ADVANCED

NOTE: For exercises using the Xercise Bar, the tubing may be rolled over the bar to achieve greater levels of tension. Make sure bolt in bar is tight and tubing is looped through all holes equally on both sides. Tie a knot with both loose ends of tubing for safety.

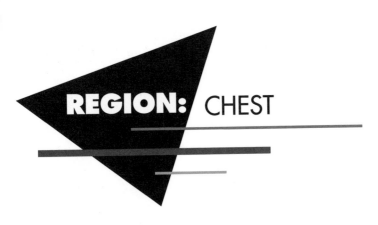

XERCISE BAR STANDING CHEST PRESS
(Pectorals)

A. Secure tubing behind middle back. Roll tubing over bar as many times as needed for proper tension.

B. Assume a square stance slightly wider than shoulder width and soften knees. Keep the hips back, pelvis tilted slightly anterior and lumbar spine neutral.

C. Grasp bar with a moderate overhand grip. The upper and lower arms should form 90° angles as the bar rests against the lower sternum.

D. With firm wrists, press out and slightly up, finishing with arms straight out from shoulders.

E. Keep the chest up, rib cage lifted, bellybutton drawn toward spine and the lumbar spine in its neutral curvature.

> **TECH TIPS**
> **This exercise may also be performed by anchoring tubing at chest height. Face away from the insertion in a square stance and perform steps C through E.**

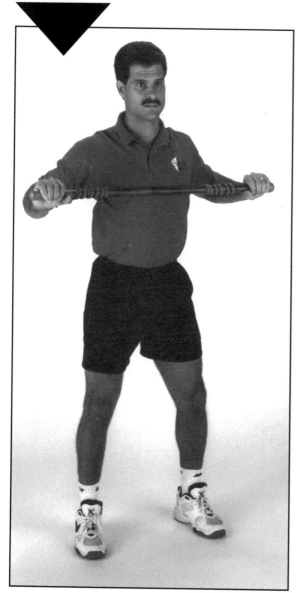

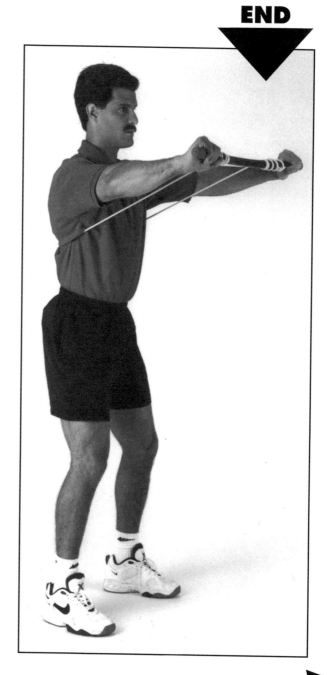

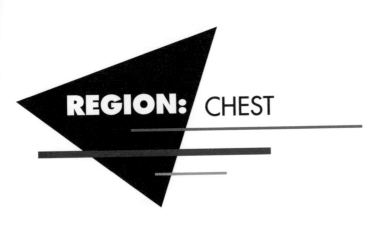

STEP XERCISE BAR SEATED CHEST PRESS

(Pectorals)

A. Tubing is secured through step strap at outside attachment.

B. Grasp bar and sit at end of step nearest to step strap.

C. Face away from attachment so that tubing pulls from behind body and place feet comfortably on floor. Roll tubing over bar as many times as needed for proper tension.

D. Hold bar with a moderate overhand grip. The upper and lower arms should form 90° angles as bar rests against lower sternum.

E. With firm wrists, press out and slightly up, finishing with arms straight out from shoulders.

F. Keep the chest up, rib cage lifted, bellybutton drawn toward spine and the lumbar spine in its neutral curvature.

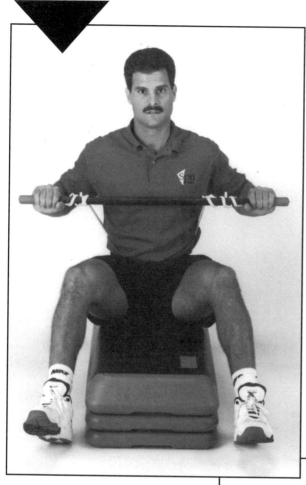

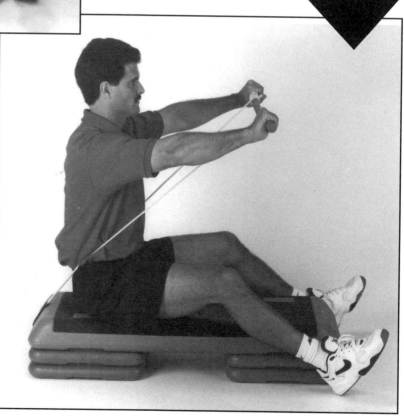

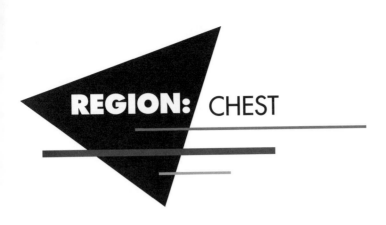

STEP XERCISE BAR SUPINE CHEST PRESS
(Pectorals)

A. Tubing is secured through step strap at inside attachment.

B. Grasp bar and lie on back with head resting comfortably at end of step nearest to step strap.

C. Place feet on step or on floor with ankles under knees. Roll tubing over bar as many times as needed for proper tension.

D. Hold bar with a moderate overhand grip. The upper and lower arms should form 90° angles as bar rests against lower sternum. The tubing attachment should be directly under the lower sternum.

E. With firm wrists, press up and slightly back, finishing with arms straight over shoulders.

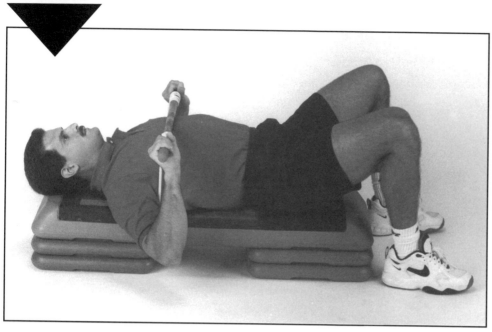

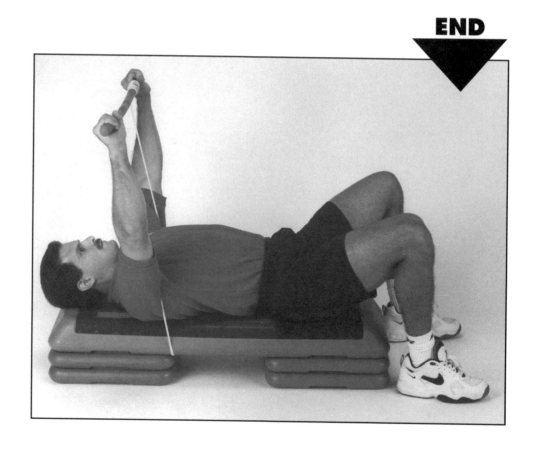

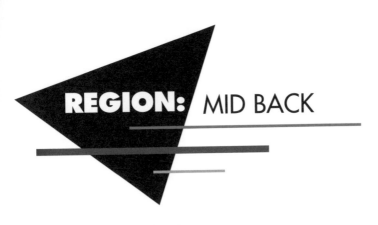

XERCISE BAR SEATED ROW (HIGH ROW OR LOW ROW)

(Middle Trapezius/Rhomboids/Latissimus Dorsi/Posterior Deltoid)

A. Sit with knees comfortably bent, center tubing under middle of both feet. Grasp tubing in between both feet and pull toward you to create a loop. Place loop back over feet.

B. Keep feet together for less resistance and apart for more resistance. Roll tubing over bar as many times as needed for proper tension.

C. Grasp bar with a moderate overhand grip (high row) or underhand grip (low row). Sit up with a slight lean forward, keeping a natural arch in lower back. Arms should be fully extended.

D. HIGH ROW - With firm wrists, bends elbows and pull Xercise Bar up and back until bar contacts upper abdomen. Elbows finish just below shoulder height with upper and lower arms forming 90° angles and shoulders abducted approximately 75°.

LOW ROW - With firm wrists, bend elbows and pull Xercise Bar back until bar contacts naval area. Elbows finish behind torso with wrists aligned with elbows and shoulders abducted approximately 30°.

E. Finish with chest expanded, rib cage lifted, shoulders over hips, lumbar spine neutral, bellybutton toward spine and shoulder blades should be squeezed back and together.

TECH TIPS

The Latissimus Dorsi is utilized to a higher degree when performing the low row (increased shoulder extension).

This exercise may also be performed by anchoring tubing at chest height. Stand in a narrow lunge position and perform steps C through E.

This exercise may also be performed by anchoring tubing at ankle height. Sit with knees comfortably bent and perform steps C through E.

The Rhomboids and Middle Trapezius are utilized to a higher degree when performing the high row (shoulder horizontal abduction).

START HIGH ROW

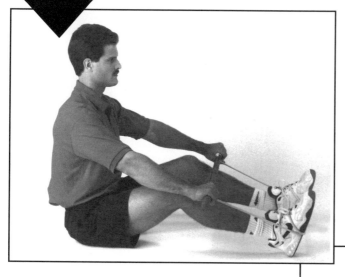

HIGH ROW **END**

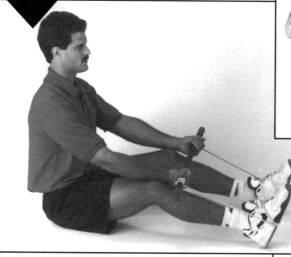

START LOW ROW

LOW ROW **END**

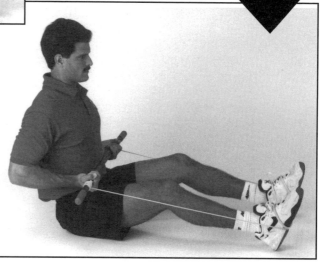

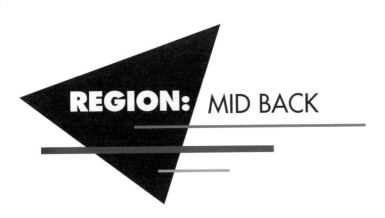

STEP XERCISE BAR SEATED ROW
(HIGH ROW OR LOW ROW)

(Middle Trapezius/Rhomboids/Latissimus Dorsi/Posterior Deltoid)

A. Tubing is secured through step strap at outside attachment.

B. Grasp bar and sit at end of step farthest from step strap.

C. Face attachment, bend knees and place heels comfortably on floor as shown.

D. Hold bar with a moderate overhand grip (high row) or underhand grip (low row). Sit up with a slight lean forward, keeping a natural arch in lower back. Arms should be fully extended.

E. **HIGH ROW -** With firm wrists, bend elbows and pull Xercise Bar up and back until bar contacts upper abdomen. Elbows finish just below shoulder height with upper and lower arms forming 90° angles and shoulders abducted approximately 75°.

LOW ROW - With firm wrists, bend elbows and pull Xercise Bar back until bar contacts naval area. Elbows finish behind torso with wrists aligned with elbows and shoulders abducted approximately 30°.

F. Finish with chest expanded, rib cage lifted, shoulders over hips, lumbar spine neutral, belly-button drawn toward spine and shoulder blades should be squeezed back and together.

> **TECH TIPS**
>
> The Latissimus Dorsi is utilized to a higher degree when performing the low row (increased shoulder extension).
>
> The Rhomboids and Middle Trapezius are utilized to a higher degree when performing the high row (shoulder horizontal abduction).

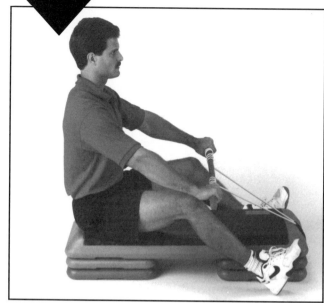

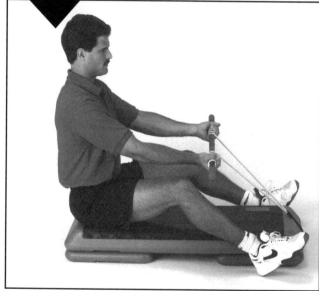

END

HIGH ROW

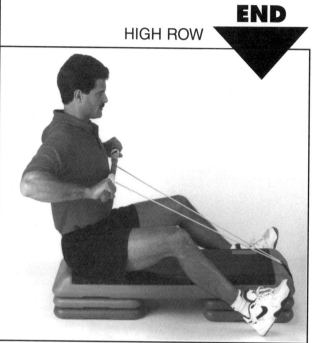

LOW ROW **END**

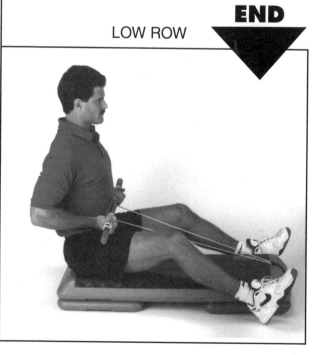

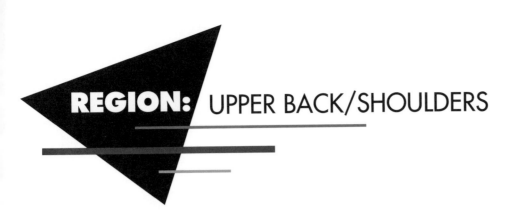

XERCISE BAR STANDING MILITARY PRESS

(Upper Trapezius/Anterior Deltoid/Medial Deltoid)

A. Stand in a narrow, staggered lunge or square stance. Place tube under arch of front foot or both feet and soften knees. Keep hips back, pelvis tilted slightly anterior and lumbar spine neutral. Roll tubing over bar as many times as needed for proper tension.

B. Grasp bar with a moderate overhead grip and place under chin on upper chest.

C. With firm wrists, press upward and finish with bar directly over shoulders.

D. Keep the chest up, rib cage lifted, bellybutton drawn toward spine and the lumbar spine in its neutral curvature.

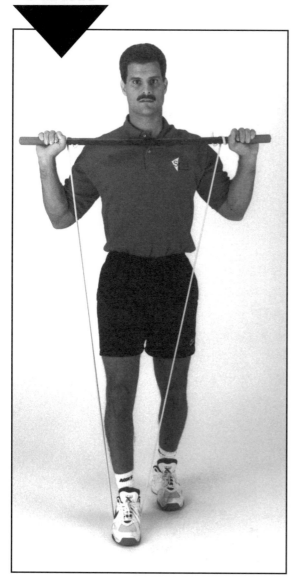

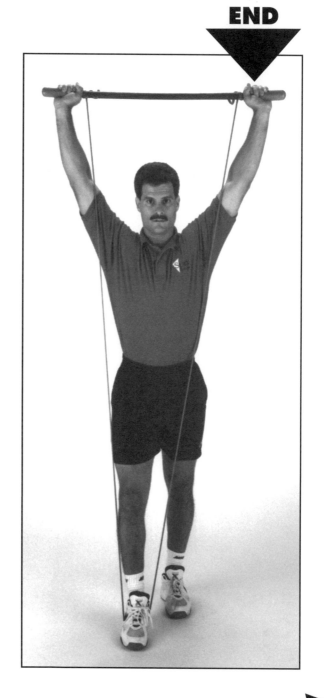

XERCISE BAR STANDING UPRIGHT ROW
(Upper Trapezius/Medial Deltoid)

A. Stand in a staggered, narrow or square stance. Place tubing under arch of front foot or both feet and soften knees. Keep hips back, pelvis tilted slightly anterior and lumbar spine neutral. Roll tubing over bar as many times as needed for proper tension.

B. Grasp bar with a moderate overhand grip allowing arms to hang straight down from shoulders. To increase upper trapezius recruitment, perform a modified shrug (scapular elevation).

C. Bend and flare elbows and immediately face palms toward floor. Hands are kept at elbow height as elbows move away from sides of body. Upper and lower arms move as one unit and wrists remain firm.

D. End with upper and lower arms forming 90° angles. Elbows should be at same height as hands and parallel to shoulders.

E. Keep the chest up, rib cage lifted, bellybutton drawn toward spine and the lumbar spine in its neutral curvature.

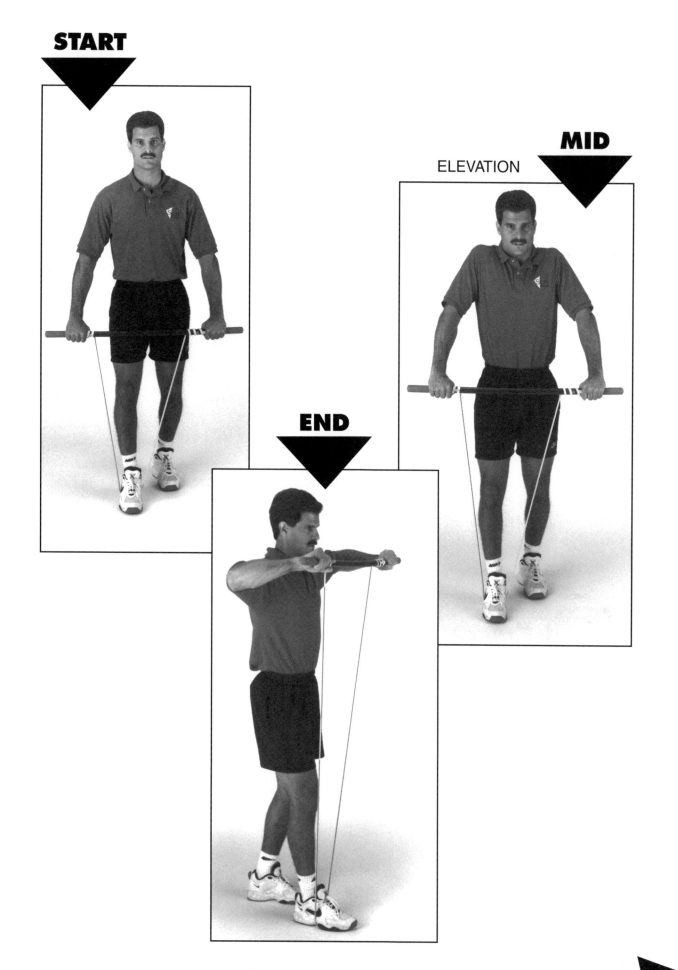

START

MID

ELEVATION

END

XERCISE BAR STANDING BEHIND BACK SHRUG

(Upper Trapezius)

A. Stand in a square stance slightly wider than shoulder width and place tubing under arches of both feet. Soften knees, keep hips back, pelvis tilted slightly anterior and lumbar spine neutral.

B. Position bar behind body and with an overhand grip grasp bar approximately 30° outside hip width.

C. Roll tubing over bar as many times as needed for proper tension.

D. Push bar back slightly to clear buttocks and shrug shoulders straight upward toward ears.

E. Keep the chest up, rib cage lifted, bellybutton drawn toward spine and the lumbar spine in its neutral curvature.

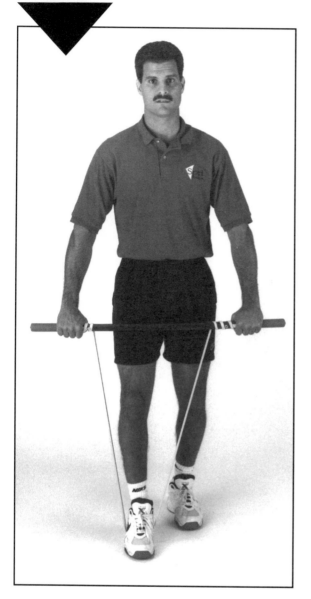

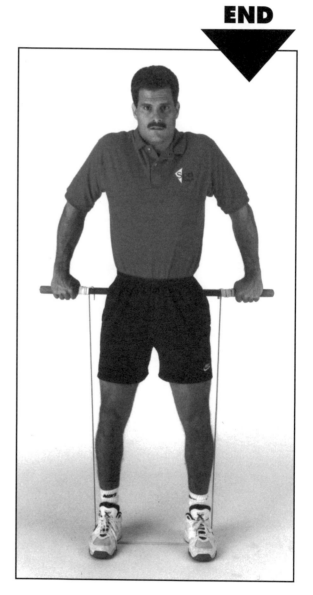

STEP XERCISE BAR STANDING MILITARY PRESS

(Upper Trapezius/Anterior Deltoid/Medial Deltoid)

A. Tubing is secured through step strap at outside attachment.

B. Grasp bar and stand at end of step nearest to step strap.

C. Face away from attachment in a narrow, staggered lunge position. Soften knees, keep hips back, pelvis tilted slightly anterior and lumbar spine neutral.

D. Hold bar with a moderate overhead grip and place under chin on upper chest.

E. With firm wrists, press upward and finish with bar directly over shoulders.

F. Keep the chest up, rib cage lifted, bellybutton drawn toward spine and the lumbar spine in its neutral curvature.

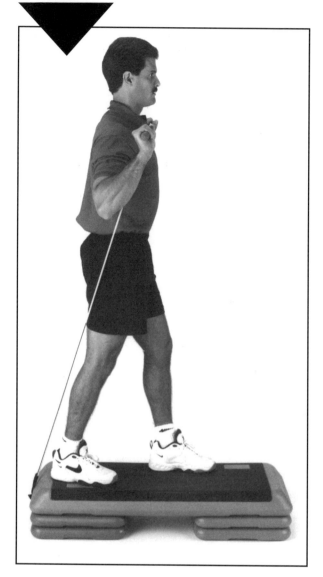

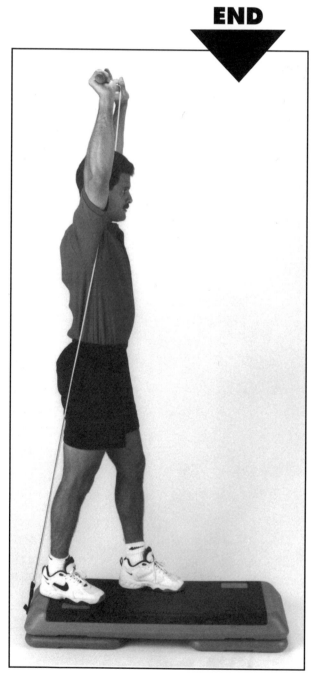

STEP XERCISE BAR STANDING UPRIGHT ROW

(Upper Trapezius/Medial Deltoid)

A. Tubing is secured through step strap at outside attachment.

B. Grasp bar and stand at end of step nearest to step strap.

C. Face attachment in a square stance. Soften knees, keep hips back, pelvis tilted slightly anterior and lumbar spine neutral.

D. Hold bar with a moderate overhand grip, allowing arms to hang straight down from shoulders. To increase upper trapezius recruitment, perform a modified shrug (scapular elevation).

E. Bend and flare elbows and immediately face palms toward floor. Hands are kept at elbow height as they are moved away from sides of body. Upper and lower arms move as one unit and wrists remain firm.

F. End with upper and lower arms forming 90° angles. Elbows should be at same height as hands and parallel to shoulders.

G. Keep the chest up, rib cage lifted, bellybutton drawn toward spine and the lumbar spine in its neutral curvature.

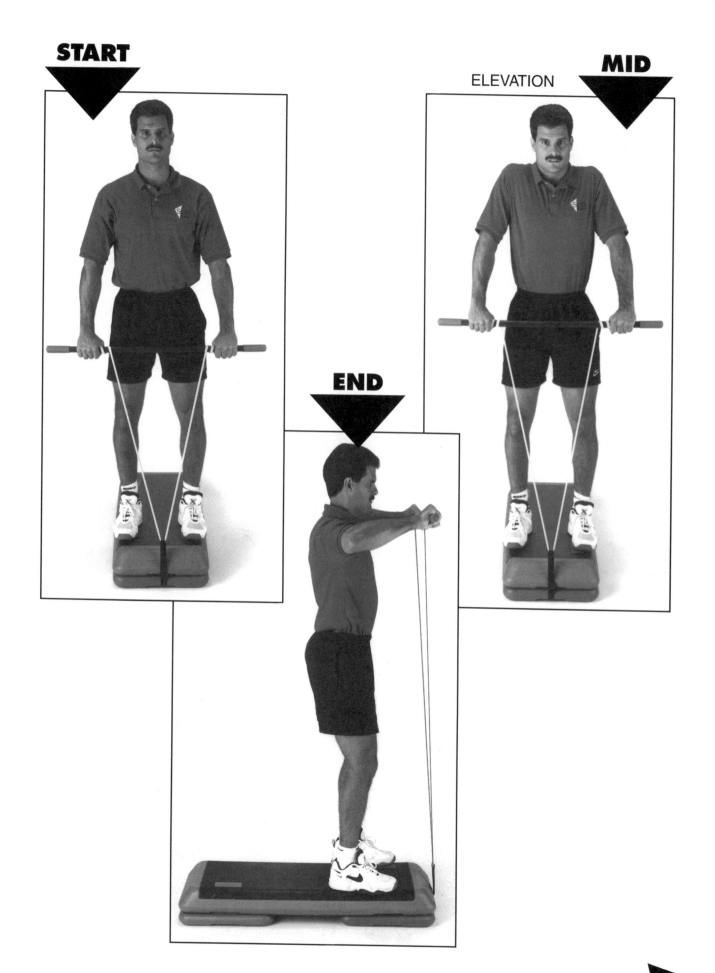

START

MID

ELEVATION

END

STEP XERCISE BAR STANDING BEHIND BACK SHRUG

(Upper Trapezius)

A. Tubing is secured through step strap at outside attachment.

B. Grasp bar and stand in a square stance at end of step nearest to step strap. Soften knees, keep hips back, pelvis tilted slightly anterior and lumbar spine neutral.

C. Face away from attachment so that tubing pulls from behind body.

D. Position bar behind body and with an overhand grip, grasp approximately 30° outside hip width.

E. Roll tubing over bar as many times as needed for proper tension.

F. Push bar back slightly to clear buttocks and shrug shoulders straight upward towards ears.

G. Keep the chest up, rib cage lifted, bellybutton drawn toward spine and the lumbar spine in its neutral curvature.

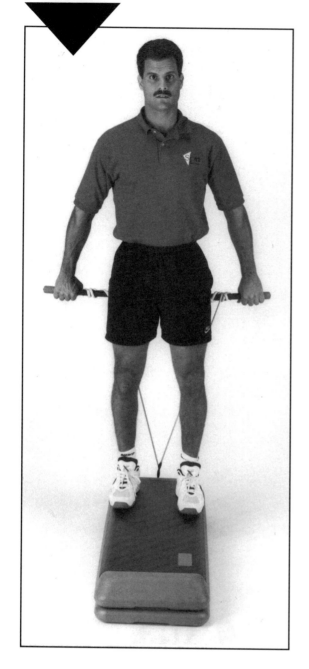

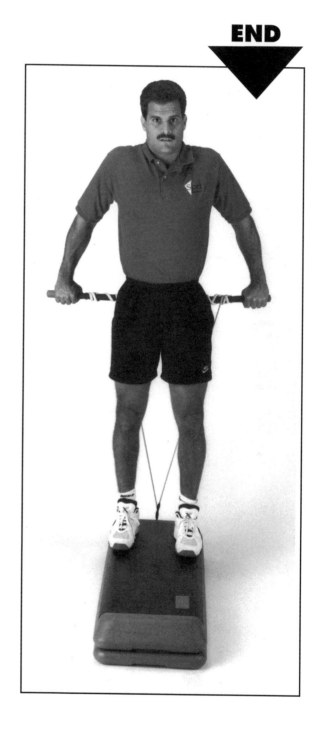

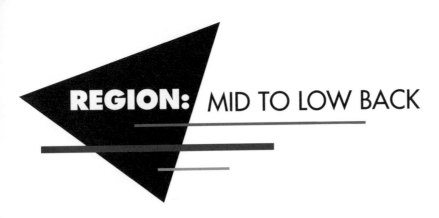

XERCISE BAR STANDING STRAIGHT ARM PULL DOWN

(Latissimus Dorsi/Lower Trapezius)

A. Anchor tubing just above head height. Place palms of open hands on Xercise Bar in a moderate overhand position (cupped grip). Back away from insertion until arms fully lengthen.

B. Assume a square stance slightly wider than shoulder width. Extend hips back, soften knees, tilt pelvis slightly anterior and draw bellybutton toward spine. Roll tubing over bar as many times as needed for proper tension.

C. Start with hands just above shoulder height. From a straight arm and stiff wrist position, press downward until palms touch thighs. Hands will finish under shoulders.

D. End with chest expanded, rib cage lifted, lumbar spine neutral and shoulder blades pulled down, back and together.

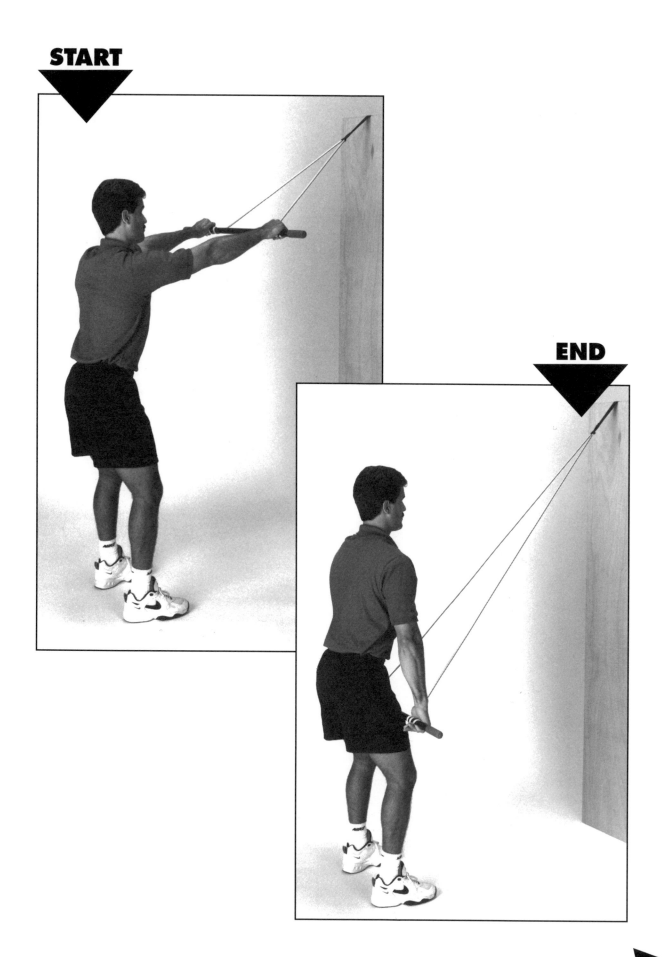

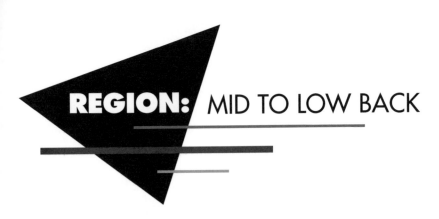

XERCISE BAR KNEELING OR SEATED FRONT PULL DOWN

(Latissimus Dorsi/Lower Trapezius)

A. Anchor tubing above head height. Roll tubing over bar as many times as needed for proper tension.

B. Sit or kneel in a staggered lunge position and grasp bar with an overhand grip one to two hands outside shoulder width.

C. Bend and flare elbows away from sides of body while pulling bar to lower chest. Keep eyes on attachment site as shoulder blades are squeezed down, back and together.

D. Keep the chest up, rib cage lifted, bellybutton drawn toward spine and the lumbar spine in its neutral curvature.

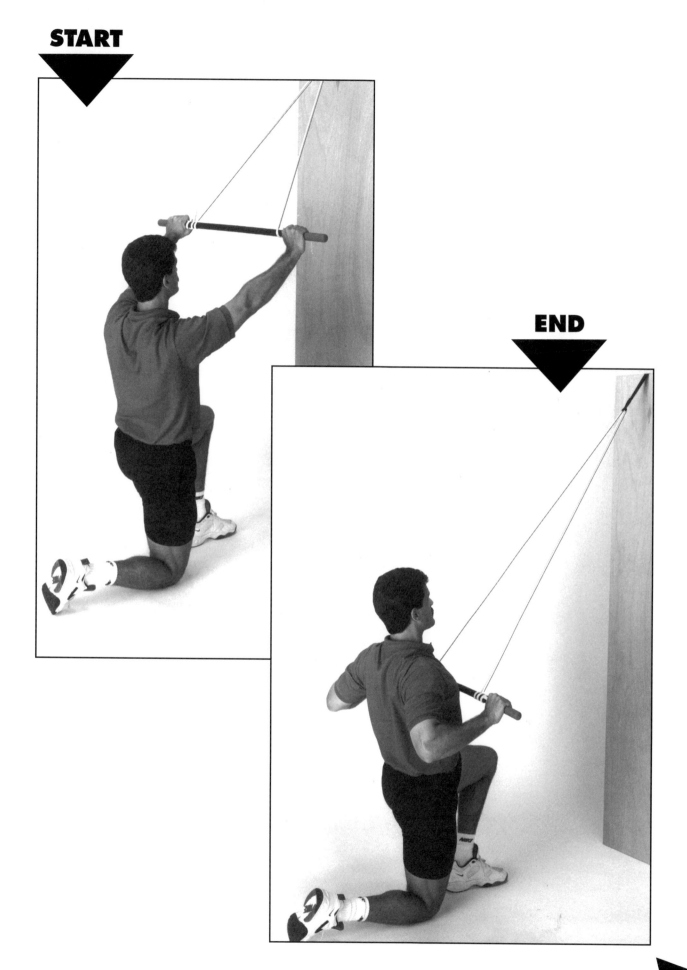

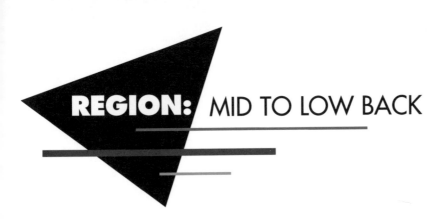
XERCISE BAR 20°-30° BENCH SUPINE STIFF ARM PULL OVER (Low Anchor)

(Latissimus Dorsi, Lower Trapezius)

A. Anchor tubing at ankle height directly in line with middle of bench. Adjust end of bench closest to attachment site to a 20°–30° angle. Move bench away from attachment site to place desired tension level on tubing once in the starting position. Lie supine with head at high end and place feet on bench with knees bent.

B. Raise hands overhead slightly wider than shoulders with palms facing up. Have partner place bar in hands. Grasp bar with an overhand grip (pronated) slightly outside shoulder width. Roll tubing over bar as many times as needed for proper tension, then position bar in the back portion of hands using a cupped grip.

C. Maintaining a stiff arm position, press upward toward ceiling, keeping wrists firm and hands open. Focus on lifting the rib cage throughout and finish with the arms straightened over the lower chest.

D. Slowly return to the starting position without allowing the hips to raise.

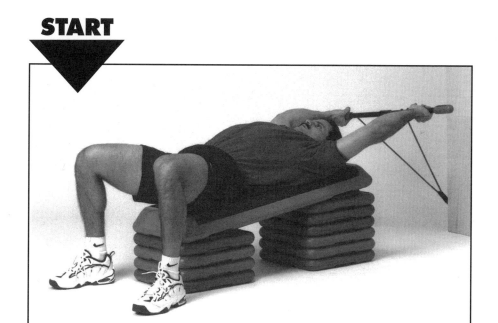

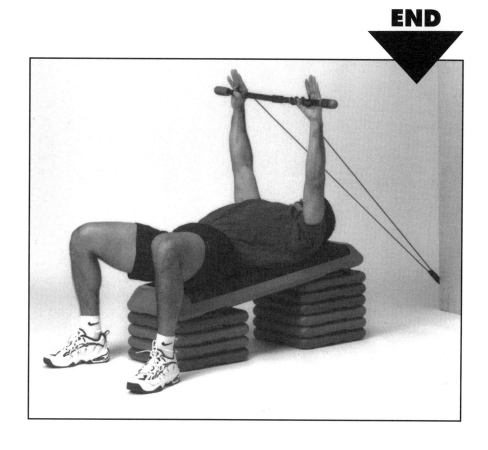

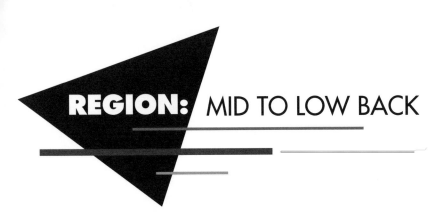

XERCISE BAR 20°-30° BENCH SUPINE STIFF ARM PULL OVER (High Anchor)

(Latissimus Dorsi, Lower Trapezius)

A. Anchor tubing at top of door directly in line with middle of bench. Adjust end of bench closest to attachment site to a 20-30° angle. Move bench away from attachment site to place desired tension level on tubing once in the starting position. Lie supine with head at high end and place feet on bench with knees bent.

B. Raise hands overhead slightly wider than shoulders with palms facing up. Have partner place bar in hands. Grasp bar with an overhand grip (pronated) slightly outside shoulder width. Roll tubing over bar as many times as needed for proper tension, then position bar in the back portion of hands using a cupped grip.

C. Maintaining a stiff arm position, press downward keeping wrists firm and hands open while expanding the chest and lifting the rib cage. Finish with the bar contacting the mid-thighs, palms facing down and slightly outside hips, shoulder blades squeezed together and bellybutton drawn toward spine.

D. Slowly return to the starting position without allowing the hips to raise.

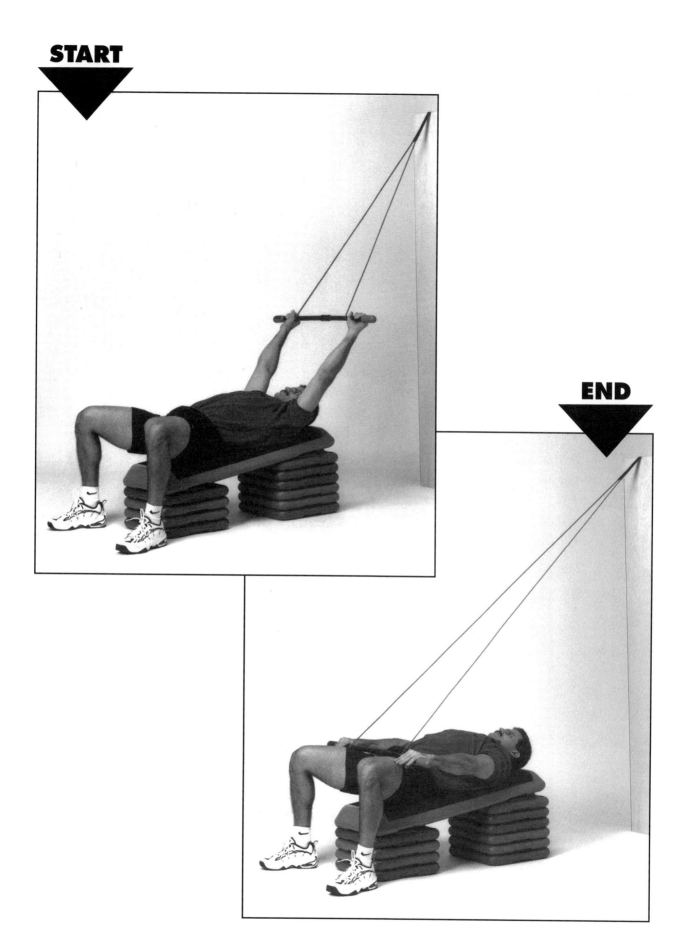

XERCISE BAR STANDING REVERSE PULL OVER

(Anterior Deltoid, Lower Trapezius)

A. Anchor tubing at ankle height with torso facing attachment site.

B. Grasp bar with an overhand grip slightly outside shoulder width. Move away from attachment site to desired tension level or roll tubing over bar as many times as needed and stand upright. Straighten arms toward knees allowing arms to hang comfortably.

C. Place feet approximately shoulder width apart. Lead with hips and perform a half-squat while keeping arms straight. With firm wrists, pull up and back keeping arms straight while simultaneously rising from the half-squat. Focus on expanding the chest, lifting the rib cage, and drawing the bellybutton toward spine.

D. Finish with the arms straightened overhead and knuckles facing ceiling. Keep the natural lumbar curvature while standing fully upright. Do not allow the pelvis to tuck under or lower spine to arch excessively.

E. Slowly return to the half–squat starting position.

START

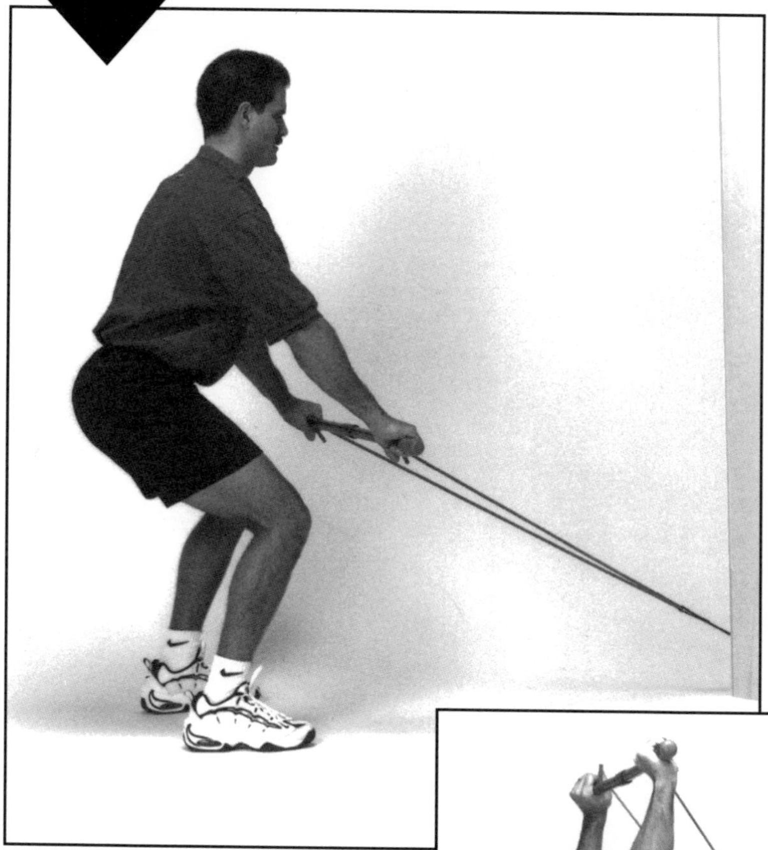

END

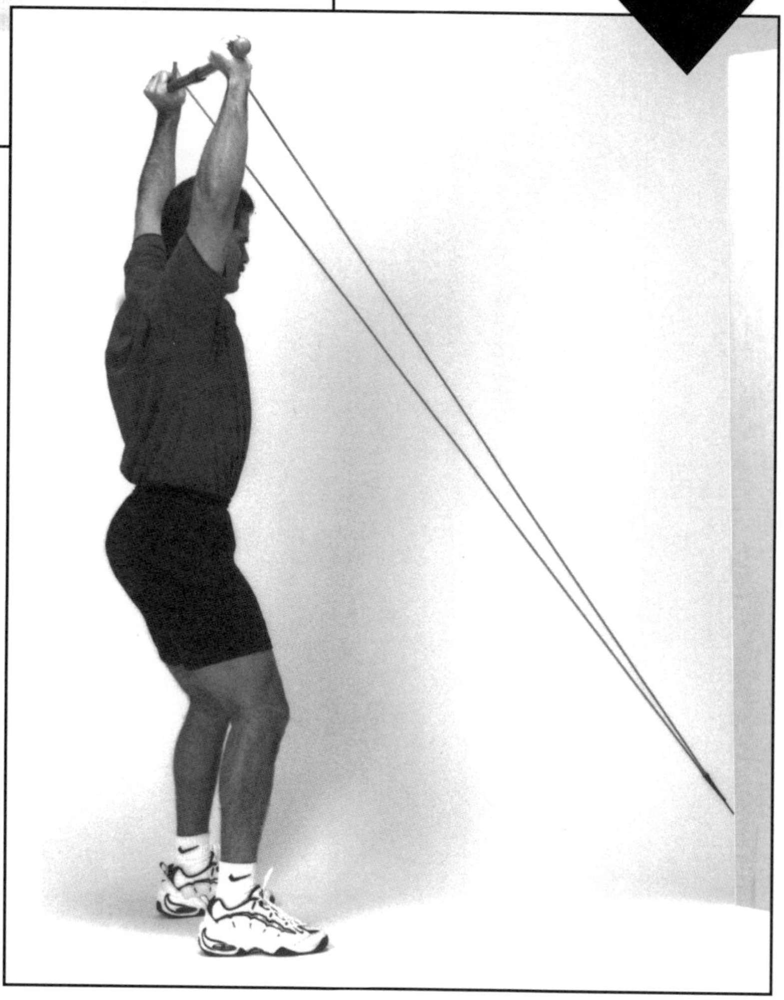

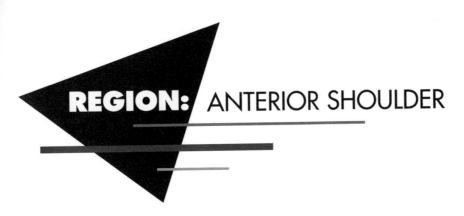

REGION: ANTERIOR SHOULDER

XERCISE BAR STANDING FRONT RAISE
(Anterior Deltoid)

A. Stand in a staggered, narrow or wide stance. Place tubing under arch of front foot or both feet and soften knees. Keep hips back, pelvis tilted slightly anterior and lumbar spine neutral.

B. Grasp bar with a moderate overhand grip with hands slightly outside shoulders and rest bar against thighs. Roll tubing over bar as many times as needed for proper tension.

C. With firm wrists, raise arms up and forward, finishing with elbows soft and at shoulder height.

D. Keep the chest up, rib cage lifted, bellybutton drawn toward spine and the lumbar spine in its neutral curvature.

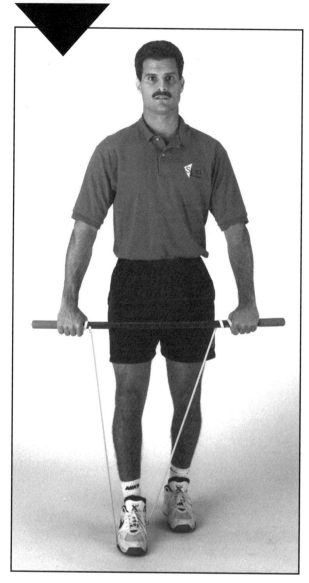

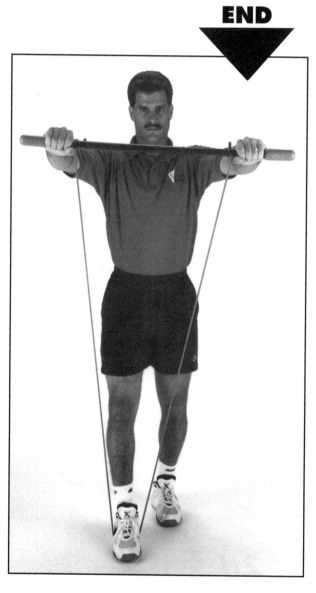

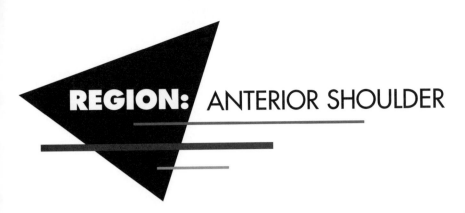

STEP XERCISE BAR STANDING FRONT RAISE

(Anterior Deltoid)

A. Tubing is secured through step strap at outside attachment.

B. Grasp bar and stand on step nearest to step strap.

C. Face attachment in a narrow, square stance. Soften knees, keep hips back, pelvis tilted slightly anterior and lumbar spine neutral.

D. Hold bar with a moderate overhand grip with hands slightly outside shoulders and rest bar against thighs. Roll tubing over bar as many times as needed for proper tension.

E. With firm wrists, raise arms up and forward, finishing with elbows soft and at shoulder height.

F. Keep the chest up, rib cage lifted, bellybutton drawn toward spine and the lumbar spine in its neutral curvature.

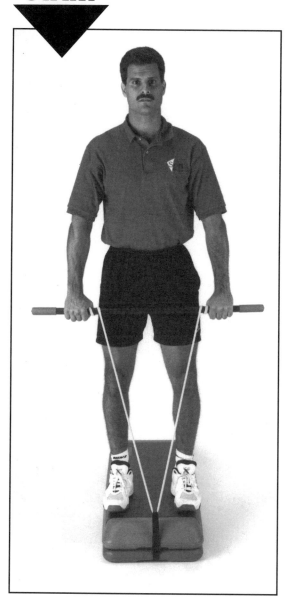

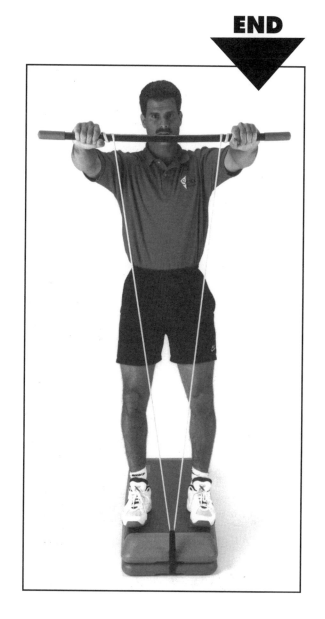

XERCISE BAR STANDING ARM CURL

(Biceps)

▼ **Position of shoulder joint - Neutral**

A. Stand in a staggered, narrow or wide stance. Place tubing under arch of front foot or both feet and soften knees. Keep hips back, pelvis tilted slightly anterior and lumbar spine neutral.

B. Grasp bar with an underhand grip and straighten arms comfortably under shoulders.

C. Roll tubing over bar as many times as needed for proper tension.

D. Bend elbows and curl fully, ending with palms facing front part of shoulders. Finish with elbows directly under shoulders.

E. Keep the chest up, rib cage lifted, bellybutton drawn toward spine and the lumbar spine in its neutral curvature.

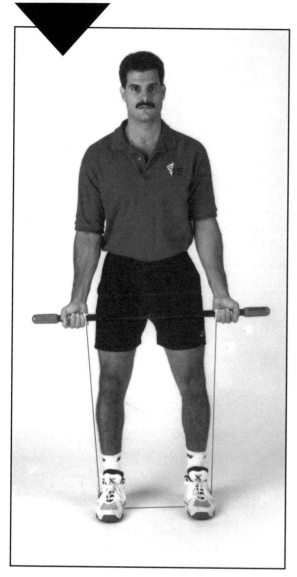

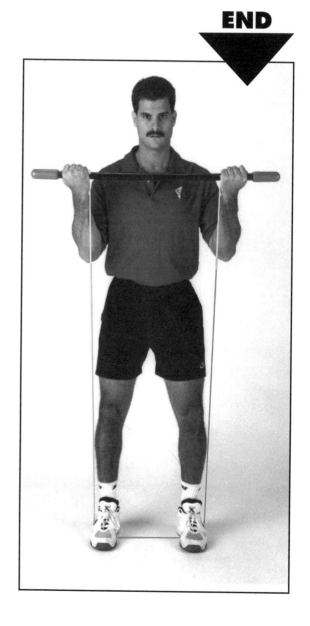

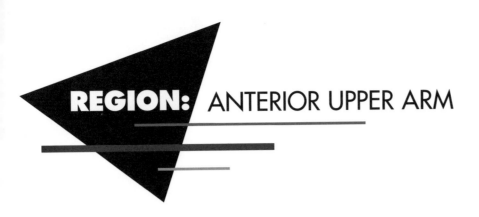

XERCISE BAR STANDING ARM CURL

(Biceps)

▼ **Position of shoulder joint - Frontal**

A. Anchor tubing at shoulder height and grasp bar with an underhand grip.

B. With hands in alignment with shoulders, back away from insertion until arms fully lengthen.

C. Roll tubing over bar as many times as needed for proper tension. Assume a square stance slightly wider than shoulder width and soften knees. Keep hips back, pelvis tilted slightly anterior and lumbar spine neutral.

D. Keep arms at shoulder height with palms of hands facing up.

E. Bend elbows and curl fully, ending with palms facing back. Finish with elbows aligned with shoulders.

F. Keep the chest up, rib cage lifted, bellybutton drawn toward spine and the lumbar spine in its neutral curvature.

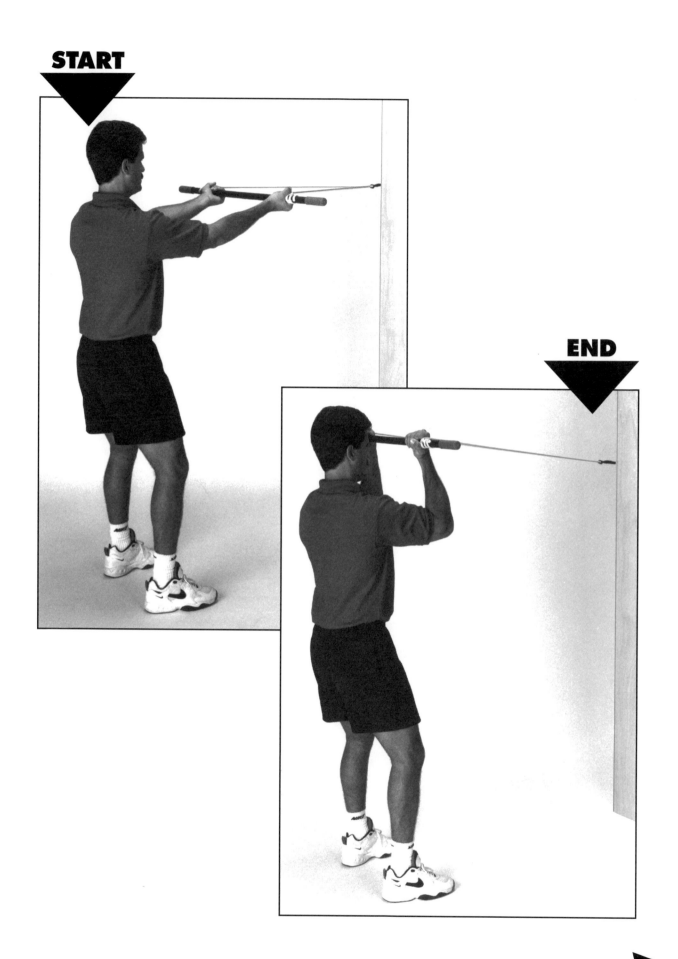

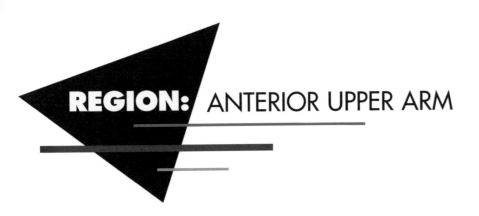

XERCISE BAR BENCH SUPINE PREACHER ARM CURL

(Biceps)

▼ Position of shoulder jont - Frontal

A. Anchor tubing at top of door directly in line with middle of bench. Move bench away from attachment site to place desired tension on tubing once in the starting position. Lie supine with head at end of bench toward attachment site. Place feet on bench with knees bent and raise hands directly over shoulders.

B. Have partner place bar in hands. Grasp bar with an overhand grip (pronated) slightly inside shoulder width. Roll tubing over bar as many times as needed for proper tension. Keep the upper arms aligned over shoulders with palms facing back.

C. With firm wrists, bend elbows and perform the curling motion while keeping the elbows and upper and lower arms stationary. Keep the chest expanded, rib cage lifted and bellybutton drawn toward spine.

D. Finish with the elbows directly over the shoulders, bar contacting the top of forehead and knuckles facing behind body.

E. Slowly return to the starting position.

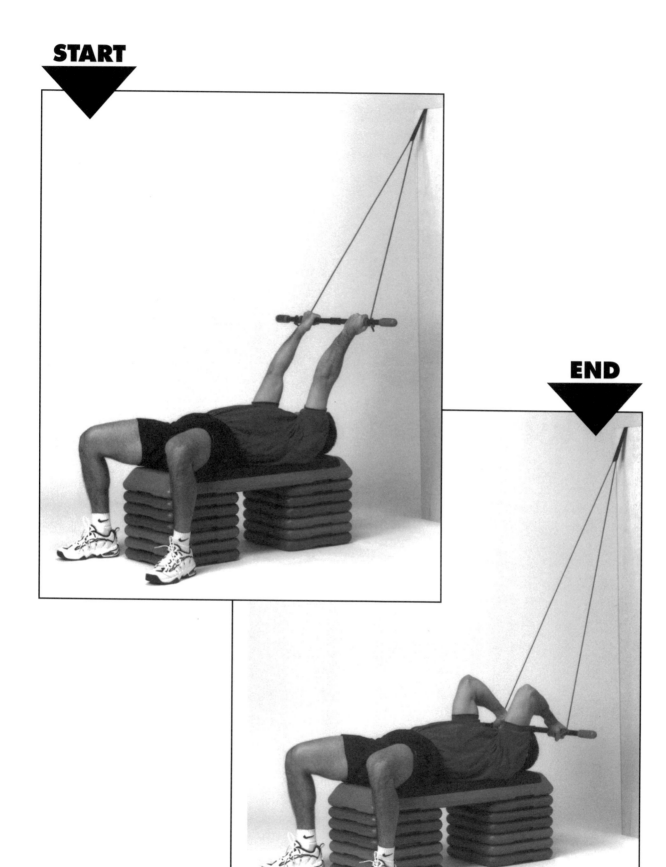

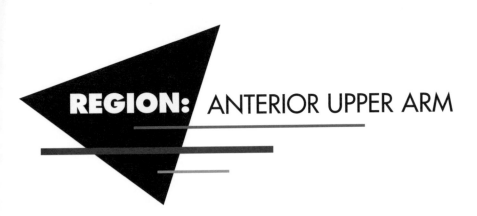

STEP XERCISE BAR STANDING ARM CURL
(Biceps)

▼ **Position of shoulder joint - Neutral**

A. Tubing is secured through step strap at outside attachment.

B. Grasp bar and stand at end of step nearest to step strap.

C. Face attachment and stand in a square stance. Soften knees, keep hips back, pelvis tilted slightly anterior and lumbar spine neutral.

D. Hold bar with an underhand grip and straighten arms comfortably under shoulders.

E. Roll tubing over bar as many times as needed for proper tension.

F. Bend elbows and curl fully, ending with palms facing front part of shoulders. Finish with elbows directly under shoulders.

G. Keep the chest up, rib cage lifted, bellybutton drawn toward spine and the lumbar spine in its neutral curvature.

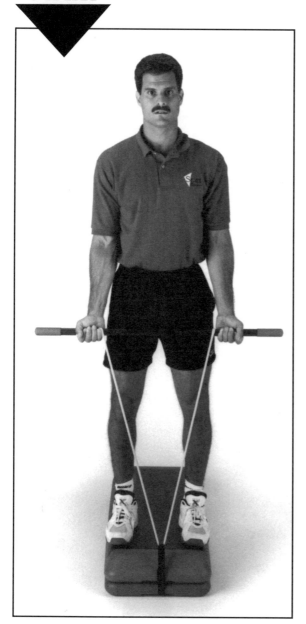

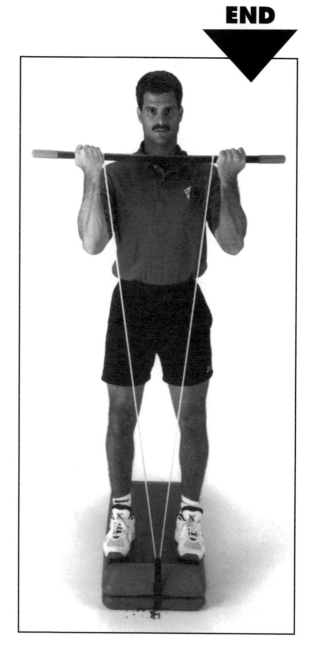

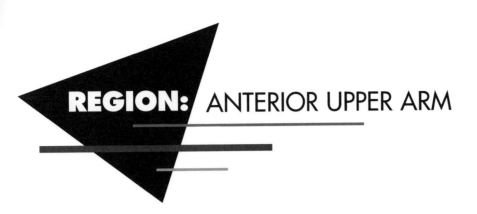

STEP XERCISE BAR SEATED ARM CURL

(Biceps)

▼ Position of shoulder joint - Frontal

A. Tubing is secured through step strap at outside attachment.

B. Grasp bar and sit on step farthest from step strap.

C. Face attachment and place heels comfortable on floor as shown.

D. Hold bar with an underhand grip. Flex shoulders 45° and straighten arms in alignment with shoulders. Roll tubing over bar as many times as needed for proper tension.

E. Bend elbows and curl fully, ending with palms facing front part of shoulders. Finish with shoulders flexed 45° and elbows aligned with shoulders.

F. Keep the chest up, rib cage lifted, bellybutton drawn toward spine and the lumbar spine in its neutral curvature.

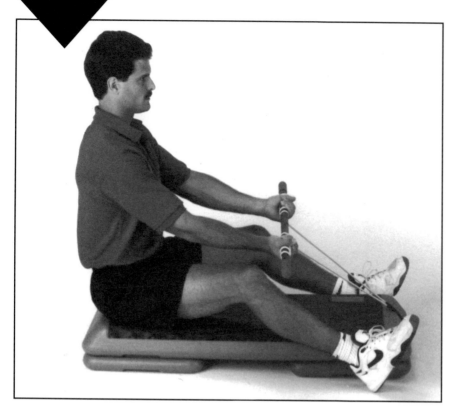

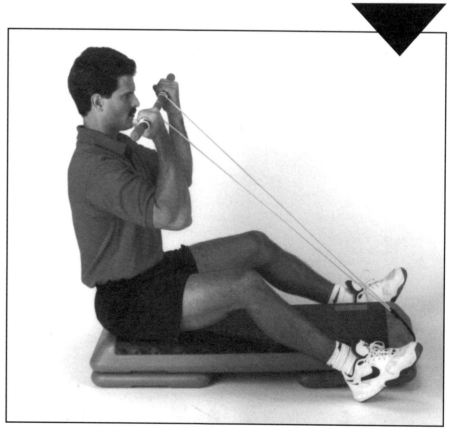

XERCISE BAR STANDING PRESS DOWN

(Triceps)

▼ Position of shoulder joint - Neutral

A. Anchor tubing above head height and grasp bar slightly inside shoulder width with an overhead grip.

B. Assume a square stance slightly wider than shoulder width and soften knees. Lean upper torso forward slightly. Keep hips back, pelvis tilted slightly anterior and lumbar spine neutral.

C. Roll tubing over bar as many times as needed for proper tension. Bend elbows and keep them directly under shoulders.

D. Hands begin slightly higher than elbows. With firm wrists, press down straightening arms fully. End with palms facing thighs, knuckles facing floor and elbows directly under shoulders.

E. Keep the chest up, rib cage lifted, bellybutton drawn toward spine and the lumbar spine in its neutral curvature.

TECH TIPS
This exercise may be performed using an underhand grip.

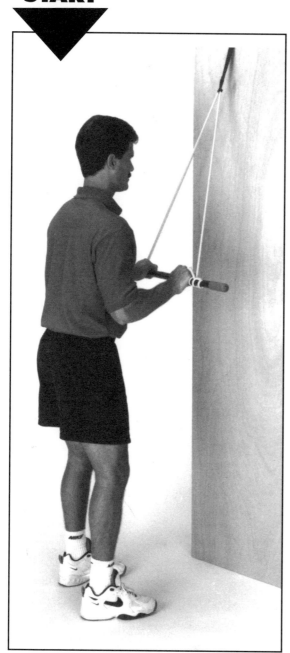

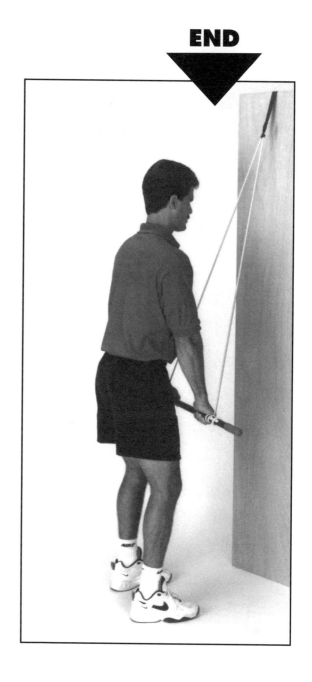

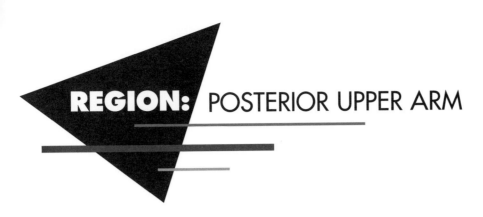

REGION: POSTERIOR UPPER ARM

XERCISE BAR STANDING OVERHEAD PRESS UP

(Triceps)

▼ Position of shoulder joint - Frontal

A. Stand in a narrow, staggered lunge stance. Position tubing under arch of rear foot and soften both knees. Keep hips back, pelvis tilted slightly anterior and lumbar spine neutral.

B. Grasp bar with an overhand grip just inside shoulder width. Roll tubing over bar as many times as needed for proper tension.

C. Raise elbows directly above shoulders and place bar along back of neck.

D. With firm wrists, press up straightening arms fully. End with hands directly over shoulders and palms facing forward with knuckles facing ceiling.

E. Keep the chest up, rib cage lifted, bellybutton drawn toward spine and the lumbar spine in its neutral curvature.

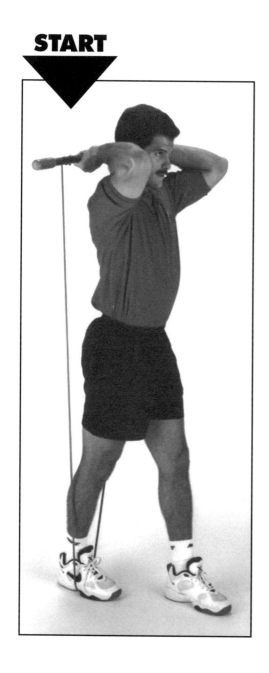

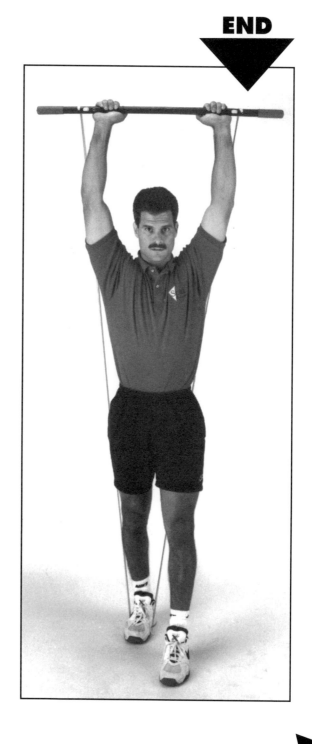

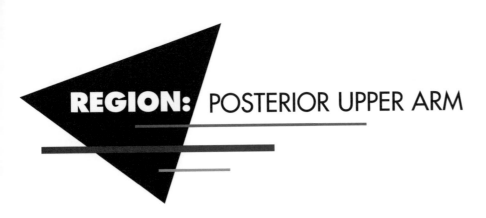

REGION: POSTERIOR UPPER ARM

XERCISE BAR STANDING PRESS OUT

(Triceps)

▼ Position of shoulder joint - Frontal

A. Anchor tubing above head height. Grasp bar slightly inside shoulder width with an overhead grip.

B. Face away from tubing attachment so it pulls from behind. Stand in a narrow, staggered lunge stance and soften both knees. Keep hips back, pelvis tilted slightly anterior and lumbar spine neutral

C. Roll tubing over bar as many times as needed for proper tension.

D. Bend arms and position elbows directly in front of shoulders with upper arms parallel to floor. Position bar over crown of head with palms facing up.

E. Lean slightly forward with upper torso. With firm wrists, press out straightening arms fully. End with palms facing down and hands in direct line with shoulders.

F. Keep the chest up, rib cage lifted, bellybutton drawn toward spine and the lumbar spine in its neutral curvature.

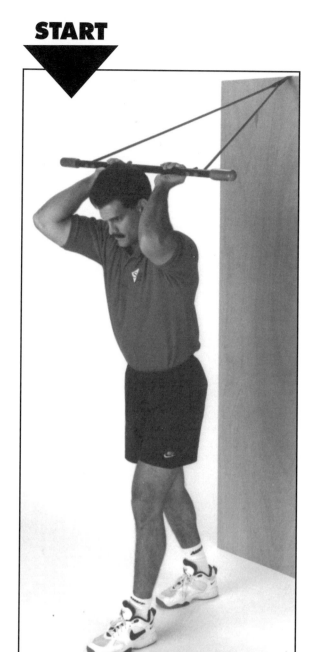

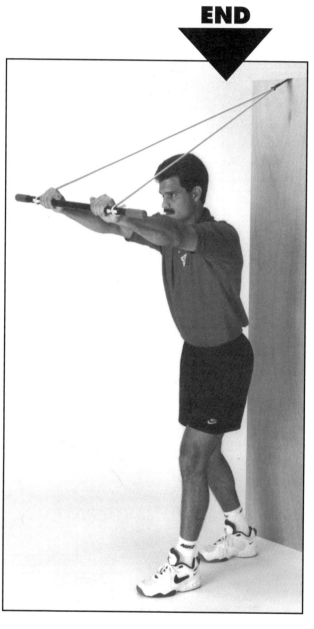

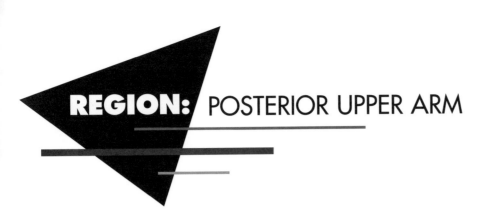

REGION: POSTERIOR UPPER ARM

XERCISE BAR BENCH SUPINE PRESS UP
(Triceps)

▼ Position of shoulder joint - Frontal

A. Anchor tubing at ankle height directly in line with middle of bench. Move bench away from attachment site to place desired tension on tubing once in the starting position. Lie supine with head at end of bench toward attachment site. Place feet on bench with knees bent and raise hands directly over shoulders with palms up.

B. Have partner place bar in hands. Grasp bar with an overhand grip (pronated) slightly inside shoulder width. Roll tubing over bar as many times as needed for proper tension. Bend elbows and position them directly over shoulders with bar contacting top of forehead.

C. With firm wrists, press upward while keeping elbows and upper and lower arms stationary. Do not allow the elbows to flare outward while pressing upward. Keep the chest expanded, rib cage lifted and bellybutton drawn toward spine.

D. Finish with the hands directly over the shoulders with knuckles facing the ceiling.

E. Slowly return to the starting position.

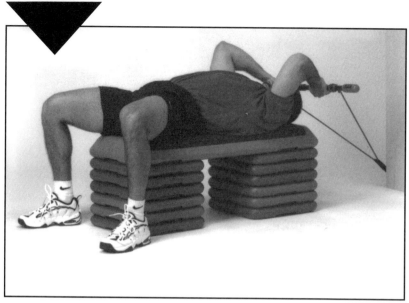

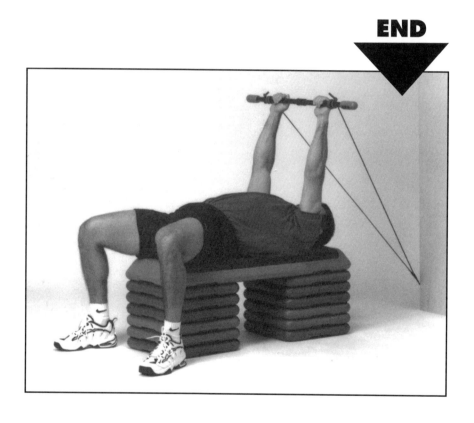

STEP XERCISE BAR STANDING OVERHEAD PRESS UP

(Triceps)

▼ Position of shoulder joint - Frontal

A. Tubing is secured through step strap at outside attachment.

B. Stand at end of step nearest to step strap.

C. Face away from attachment, in a narrow, staggered lunge position, so that tubing pulls from behind body. Soften knees, keep hips back, pelvis tilted slightly anterior and lumbar spine neutral.

D. Grasp bar with an overhand grip just inside shoulder width. Roll tubing over bar as many times as needed for proper tension.

E. Raise elbows directly above shoulders and place bar along back of neck.

F. With firm wrists, press up straightening arms fully. End with hands directly over shoulders and palms facing forward with knuckles facing ceiling.

G. Keep the chest up, rib cage lifted, bellybutton drawn toward spine and the lumbar spine in its neutral curvature.

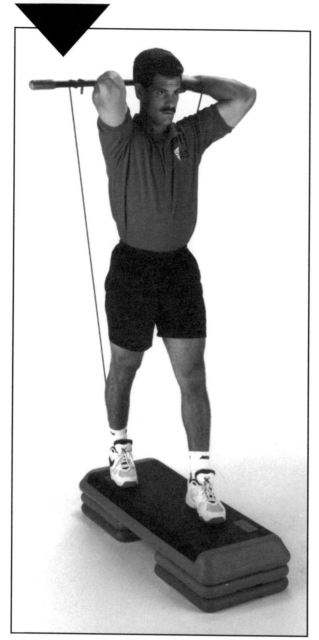

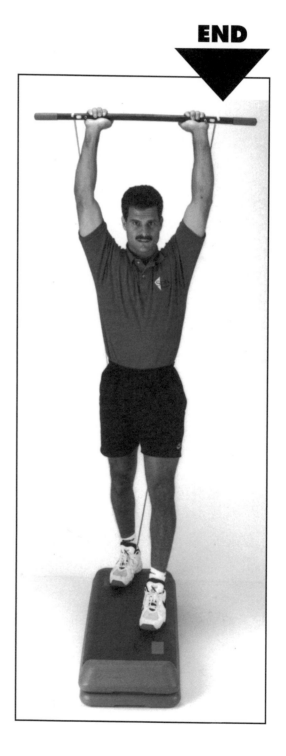

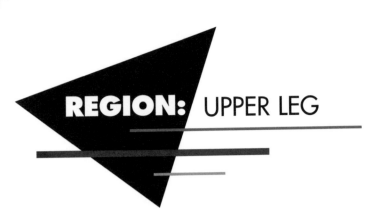

XERCISE BAR BACK SQUAT
(Quadriceps/Hamstrings/Gluteals)

A. Position feet in a moderate stance with big toes directly under hips and toes out slightly (20°–30° of external hip rotation).

B. Place tubing under arches of both feet. Grasp bar with a moderate overhand grip and rest bar on upper back over upper trapezius.

C. Keep head over hips and focus eyes slightly higher than head. Keep chest expanded, rib cage lifted, shoulder blades squeezed together and bellybutton drawn toward spine.

D. Bend knees, tilt pelvis forward (hips back) and maintain natural arch in low back. Sit back until upper legs are just above parallel in relation to floor. The lower back must maintain a neutral curvature, stop the descent when lower back loses its curvature (flexes), even if a parallel position is not achieved.

E. Keep heels down with body weight over ankles and knees over mid-foot. Middle of kneecaps align with last two toes at bottom of squat.

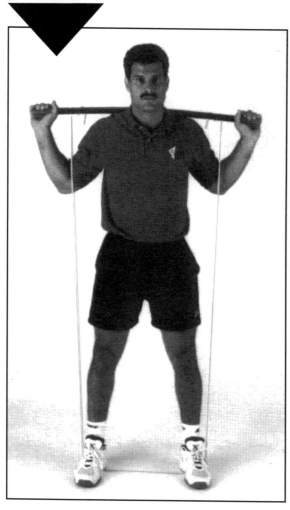

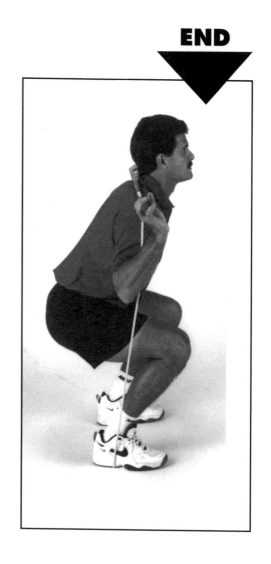

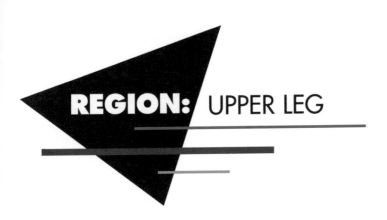

XERCISE BAR BENT TRAIL LEG LUNGE
(Quadriceps/Hamstrings/Gluteals)

A. Stand in a narrow staggered lunge stance and place tubing under arch of front foot.

B. Grasp bar with a moderate overhand grip and rest bar on upper back over upper trapezius.

C. Take a drop step with other leg and land on ball of foot. Bend knees and descend to form a 90° angle with upper and lower portion of each leg. The kneecap of lead leg should be approximately over the mid-foot. Keep heel down and weight distributed evenly through front foot. Heel of trail leg is up off floor, knee slightly behind hip and ball of foot is in contact with floor.

D. Keep head over hips and eyes focused directly forward. Keep chest expanded, rib cage lifted, shoulder blades squeezed together, bellybutton drawn toward spine and the lumber spine in its neutral curvature.

E. **STATIONARY -** Keep feet in this position, straighten both lead and trail legs simultaneously. Stand tall through ball of trail leg foot and squeeze gluteal muscles.

   DYNAMIC - Return to start position (point A) and repeat drop step (point C).

F. Place tubing under arch of other foot and repeat equal amounts of repetitions with other leg.

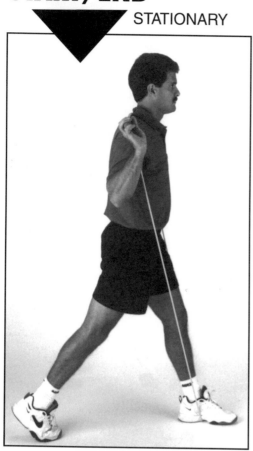

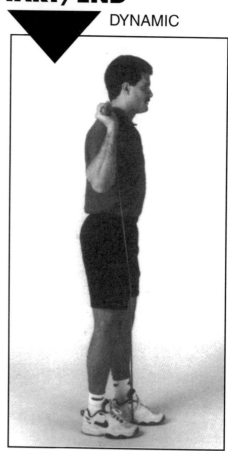

MID

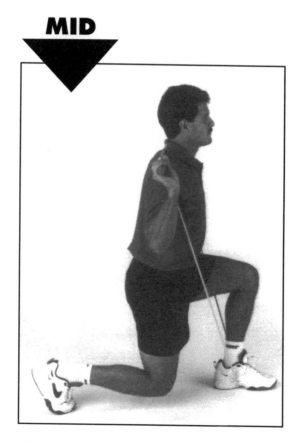

ULTRA TONER

ULTRA TONER™ RESISTANCE CHART

COLOR	RESISTANCE
PURPLE	BEGINNER
YELLOW	BEGINNER/INTERMEDIATE
GREEN	INTERMEDIATE/ADVANCED
RED	ADVANCED
BLUE	VERY ADVANCED

ANKLE WRAP

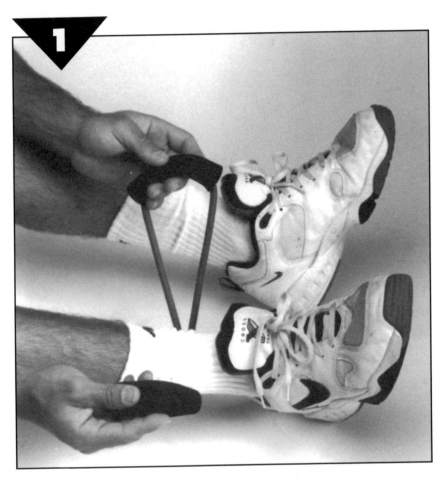

When utilizing the ankle wrap, position mid-point pad on posterior side of lower leg between calf and ankle. When using the foot wrap (not shown), place mid-point pad under arch of foot.

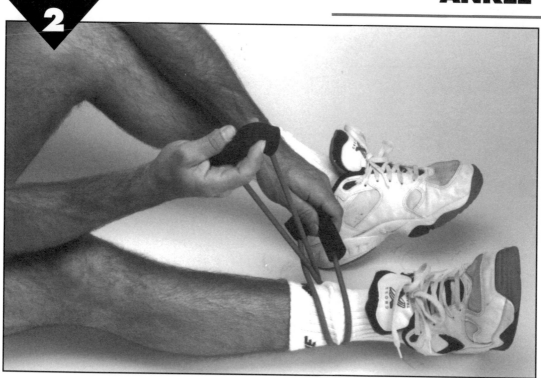

Feed handle on inside of leg through handle on outside of leg.

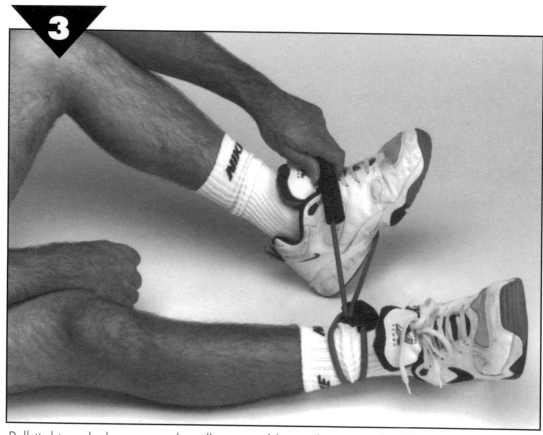

Pull tight and place open handle around lower leg or arch of foot.

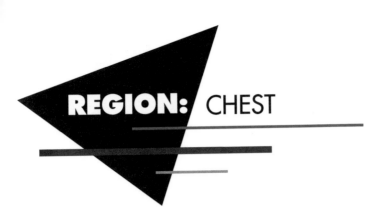

REGION: CHEST

ULTRA TONER STANDING CHEST PRESS/INCLINE PRESS

(Pectorals)

A. Secure Ultra Toner behind middle back.

B. Grasp handles and assume a square stance slightly wider than shoulder width and soften knees. Keep hips back, pelvis tilted slightly anterior and lumbar spine neutral.

C. Abduct the upper arms 30°- 45° away from torso in a thumbs up position. Elbows and wrists should be in alignment. There should be no tension in upper trapezius.

D. CHEST PRESS -
  1. With firm wrists, press out, up and together finishing in a thumbs together position (Boxers Punch) straight out from shoulders.
  2. For an advanced movement pattern, progressively rotate inward from shoulder joint ending with knuckles of index fingers together forming a V shape. Little fingers should end slightly higher than thumbs.

E. INCLINE CHEST PRESS -
  1. With firm wrists, press out, up and together finishing at eye level.
  2. For an advanced movement pattern, gradually rotate inward from shoulder joint ending with knuckles of index fingers together forming a V shape. Little fingers should end slightly higher than thumbs.

F. Keep the chest up, rib cage lifted, bellybutton drawn toward spine and the lumbar spine in its neutral curvature.

> **TECH TIPS**
> **This exercise may be performed in an alternate arm pattern.**

START

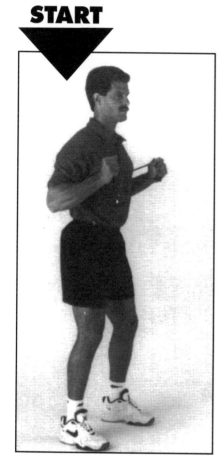

END (D1)

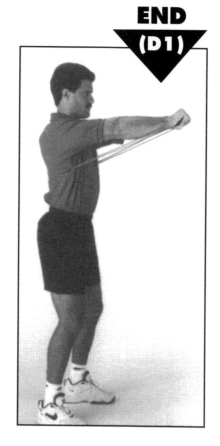

END (D2)

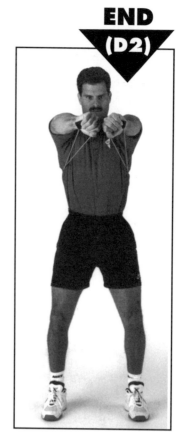

END (E1)

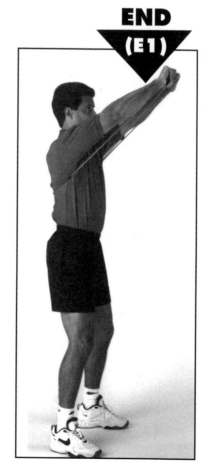

END (E2)

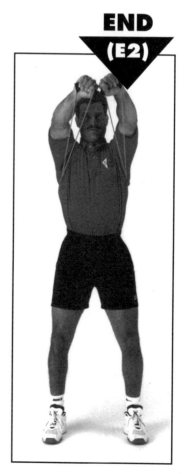

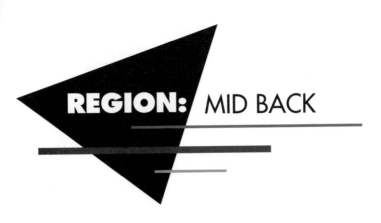

ULTRA TONER SEATED SINGLE ARM ROW (HIGH ROW OR LOW ROW)

(Middle Trapezius/Rhomboids/Latissimus Dorsi/Posterior Deltoid)

A. Sit and place one foot into one end of Ultra Toner so handle rests under arch and grasp other handle with same side hand.

B. Extend leg fully. Position exercising hand over same side knee in a palm down position. Sit up with a slight lean forward keeping a natural arch in the low back. Place other hand on opposite bent knee.

C. **HIGH ROW -** With firm wrists, bend elbow and pull hand up and back while gradually flaring elbow. Elbow finishes at shoulder height with upper and lower arm forming a 90° angle.

LOW ROW - With firm wrists, bend elbow and pull back so little finger contacts lower rib cage.

D. Finish with chest expanded, rib cage lifted, lumbar spine neutral and bellybutton drawn toward spine. Elbow finishes behind torso and shoulder blade should be squeezed toward spine.

E. Switch foot positions, place handle over foot of straightened leg and repeat equal amounts of repetitions with other hand.

> **TECH TIPS**
> The Latissimus Dorsi is utilized to a higher degree when performing the low row (increased shoulder extension).
>
> The Rhomboids and Middle Trapezius are utilized to a higher degree when performing the high row (shoulder horizontal abduction).

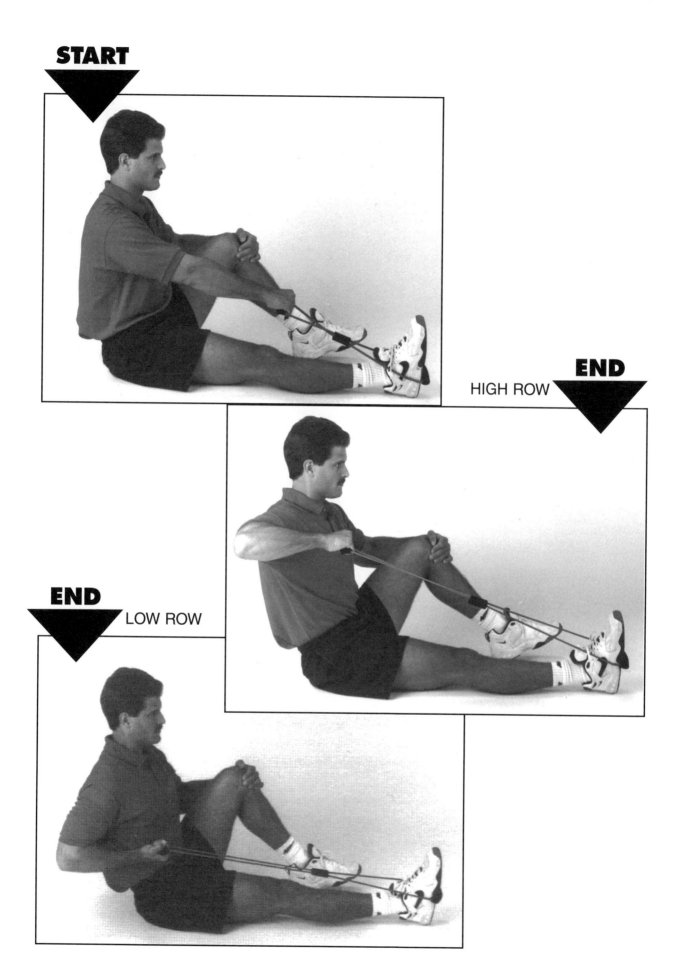

START

END
HIGH ROW

END LOW ROW

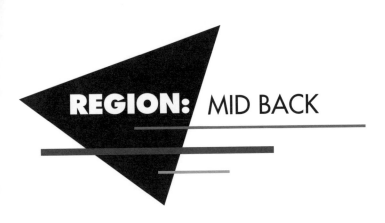

ULTRA TONER STANDING SINGLE ARM HIGH ROW

(Middle Trapezius/Rhomboids/Latissimus Dorsi/Posterior Deltoid)

A. Stand in a narrow staggered lunge position as if you were using a bow and arrow. Soften knees, keep hips back, pelvis tilted slightly anterior and lumbar spine neutral.

B. Grasp a handle with your exercising hand. With your other hand, grasp the mid-point pad, fully extend and raise arm to shoulder height in a palm down position.

C. With a firm wrist, bend elbow and pull back while gradually flaring elbow. Elbow finishes at shoulder height with upper and lower arm forming a 90° angle. The torso should rotate by one-quarter turn from midline with the shoulder blade squeezed into the spine.

D. End with chest expanded, rib cage lifted, bellybutton drawn toward spine and the lumber spine in its neutral curvature.

E. Exchange the foot and arm positions and repeat equal amounts of repetitions with other hand.

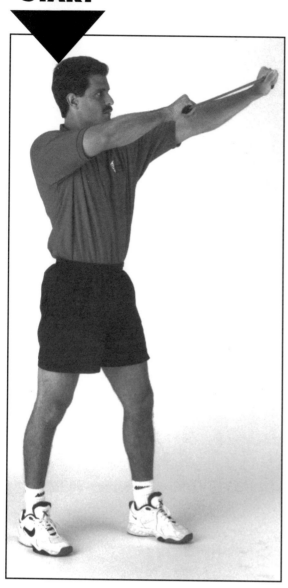

END

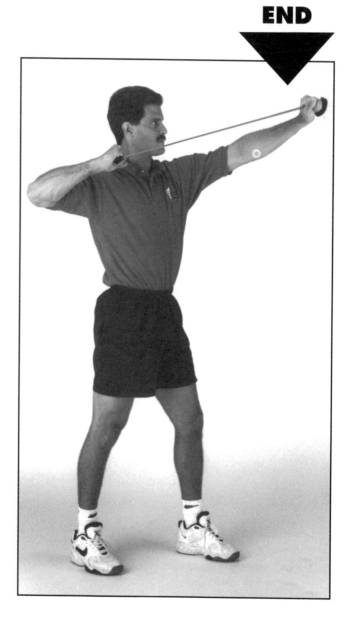

ULTRA TONER STANDING SINGLE ARM OVERHEAD PRESS

(Upper Trapezius/Anterior Deltoid/Medial Deltoid)

A. Stand in a narrow staggered lunge position. Soften knees, keep hips back, pelvis tilted slightly anterior and lumbar spine neutral.

B. Grasp a handle with your exercising hand and with your other hand grasp mid-point pad.

C. Bring exercising hand up to a comfortable position just in front of same shoulder and align opposite hand directly underneath.

D. Abduct exercising upper arm approximately 30° away from torso with thumb pointing at front portion of shoulder.

E. Press upward and back keeping wrist firm and finish with hand directly over shoulder.

F. Keep the chest up, rib cage lifted, bellybutton drawn toward spine and the lumbar spine in its neutral curvature.

G. Exchange arm positions and repeat equal amounts of repetitions with other hand.

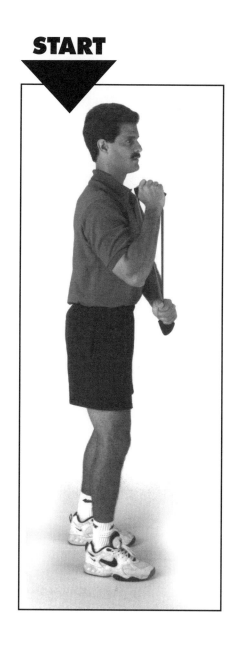

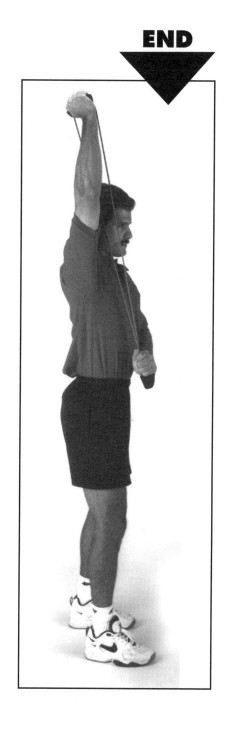

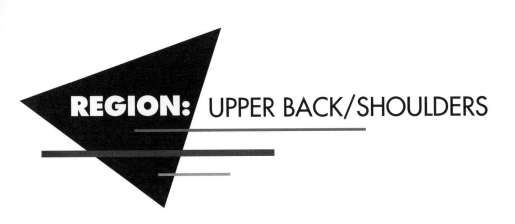

ULTRA TONER STANDING SINGLE ARM SHRUG

(Upper Trapezius/Medial Deltoid)

A. Stand and place one foot into one end of Ultra Toner so handle rests under arch.

B. Grasp other handle with your same side hand and relax arm straight down from shoulders with palm facing back.

C. Move feet just outside hip width, soften knees, keep hips back, pelvis tilted slightly anterior and lumbar spine neutral.

D. Abduct arm approximately 30° from body while shrugging shoulder straight up toward ear.

E. Keep the chest up, rib cage lifted, bellybutton drawn toward spine and the lumbar spine in its neutral curvature.

F. Place handle under other foot and repeat equal amounts of repetitions with other hand.

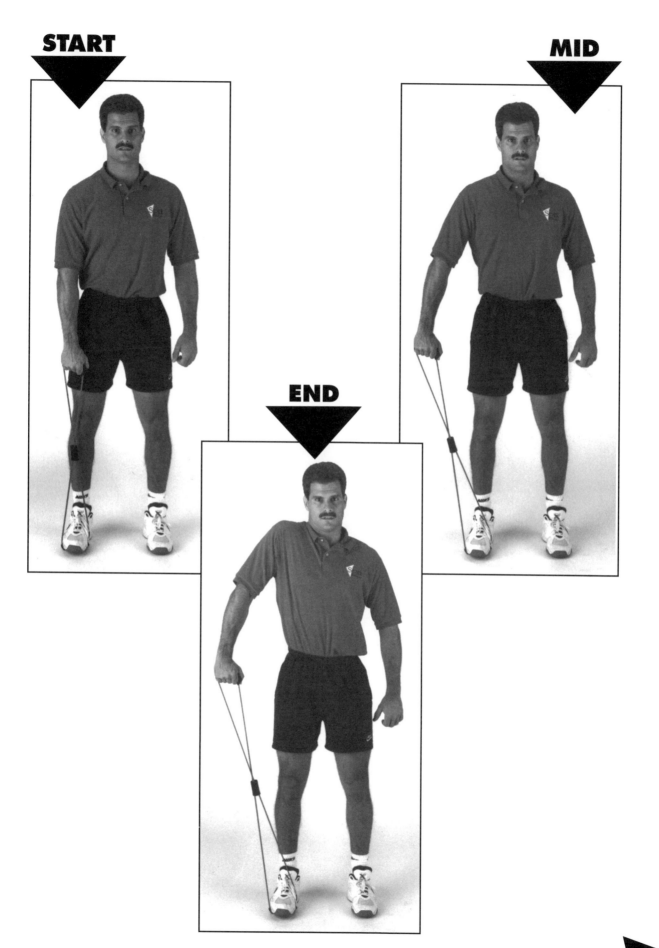

START

MID

END

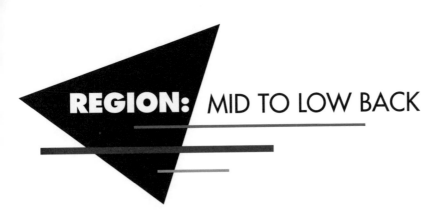

REGION: MID TO LOW BACK

ULTRA TONER STANDING SINGLE ARM PULL DOWN (HIGH PULL OR LOW PULL)

(Latissimus Dorsi/Lower Trapezius)

A. Stand in a square stance slightly wider than shoulder width and soften knees. Keep hips back, pelvis tilted slightly anterior and lumbar spine neutral.

B. Grasp a handle with your exercising hand. With your other hand, grasp mid-point pad and straighten both arms directly over shoulders.

C. Start with palms of both hands facing forward.
HIGH PULL - With a firm wrist, bend elbow and pull downward so thumb contacts outer portion of upper chest.

LOW PULL - With a firm wrist, bend elbow and pull downward so thumb contacts outer portion of lower rib cage.

D. End with chest expanded, rib cage lifted, lumbar spine neutral, bellybutton drawn toward spine, elbow pointing downward and shoulder blade squeezed toward spine.

E. Exchange arm positions and repeat equal amounts of repetitions with other hand.

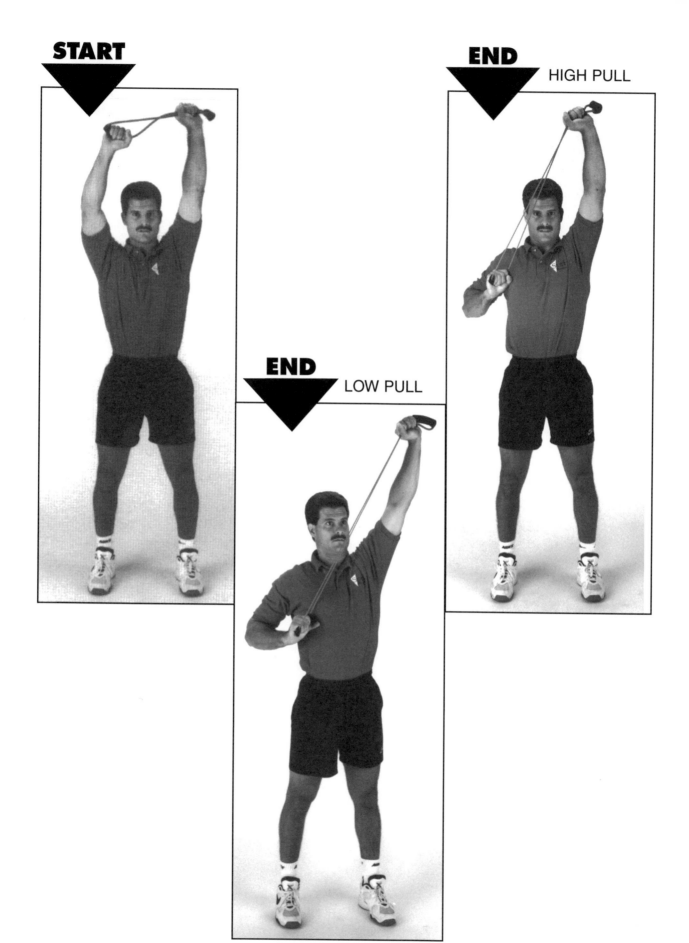

START

END HIGH PULL

END LOW PULL

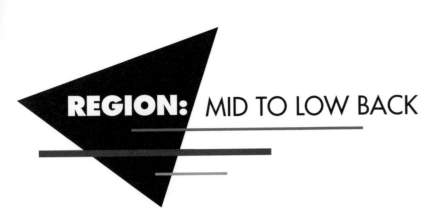

ULTRA TONER STANDING BEHIND NECK PULL DOWN

(Latissimus Dorsi/Lower Trapezius)

A. Stand in a square stance, soften knees, keep hips back, pelvis tilted slightly anterior and lumbar spine neutral. Grasp both handles with palms facing each other and raise arms directly over shoulders.

B. From straight arm position, keep wrists firm and pull down until shoulder blades are squeezed together.

C. Hands end parallel to shoulders in a thumbs up position (palms forward). Mid-point pad should be in contact with upper trapezius.

D. Keep the chest up, rib cage lifted, bellybutton drawn toward spine and the lumbar spine in its neutral curvature.

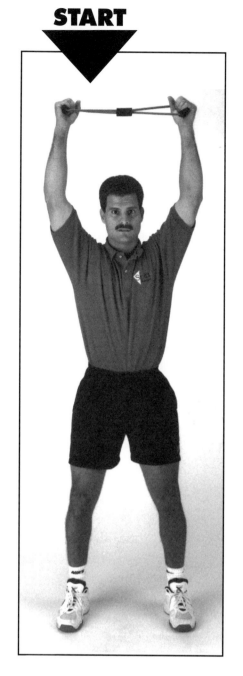

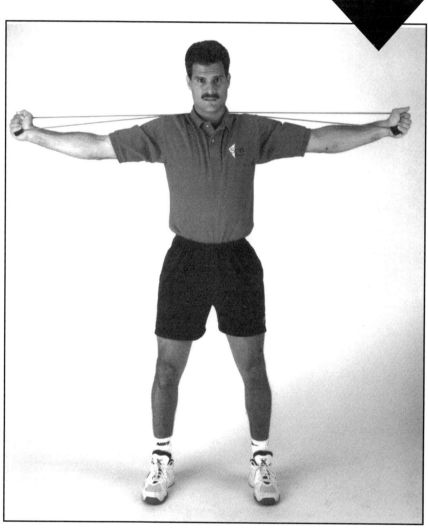

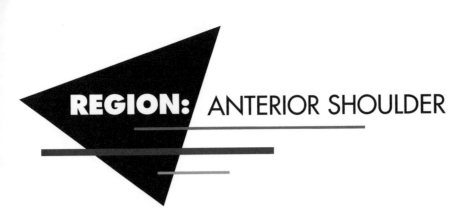

REGION: ANTERIOR SHOULDER

ULTRA TONER STANDING SINGLE ARM FRONT RAISE

(Anterior Deltoid)

A. Stand in a staggered lunge position. Soften knees, keep hips back, pelvis tilted slightly anterior and lumbar spine neutral.

B. Grasp a handle with your exercising hand. With your other hand, grasp mid-point pad, or other handle, and rest it against your opposite thigh.

C. Start with palm of exercising hand against thigh. With a firm wrist, raise arm up and forward, finishing with elbow soft and at shoulder height. Hand should end just outside shoulder width.

D. Keep the chest up, rib cage lifted, bellybutton drawn toward spine and the lumbar spine in its neutral curvature.

E. Switch arm and foot position and repeat equal amounts of repetitions with other hand.

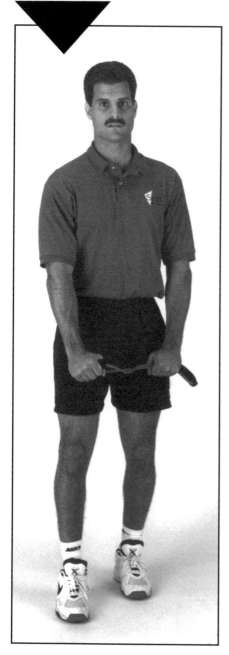

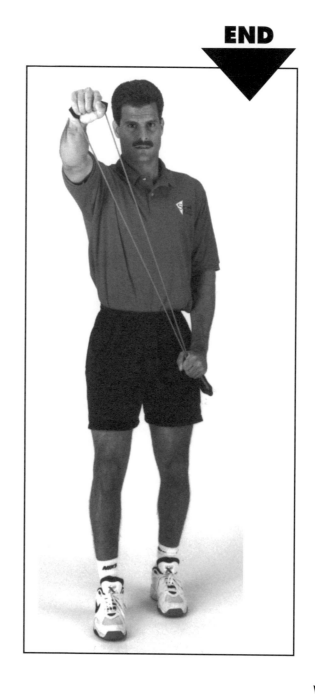

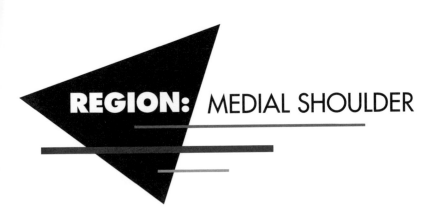

ULTRA TONER STANDING SINGLE ARM SIDE RAISE

(Medial Deltoid/External Rotators)

A. Stand in a square stance, soften knees, keep hips back, pelvis tilted slightly anterior and lumbar spine neutral.

B. Grasp a handle with your exercising hand. With your other hand, grasp mid-point pad, or other handle, and straighten directly under shoulder.

C. Place palm of exercising hand across body toward opposite hip.

D. With a firm wrist, lift arm up and away from side of body. Progressively rotate shoulder back as elbow raises to shoulder height.

E. Finish with thumb up and palm facing forward, elbow soft and in alignment with shoulder joint. Hand should be just in front of ear.

F. Keep the chest up, rib cage lifted, bellybutton drawn toward spine and the lumbar spine in its neutral curvature.

G. Switch arm and foot positions and repeat equal amounts of repetitions with other hand.

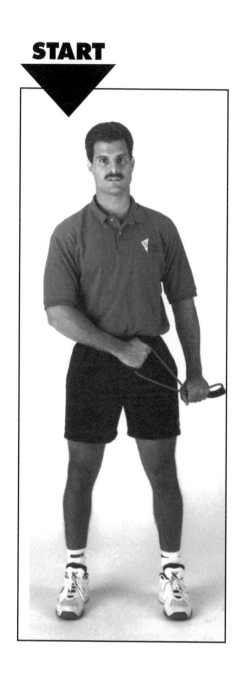

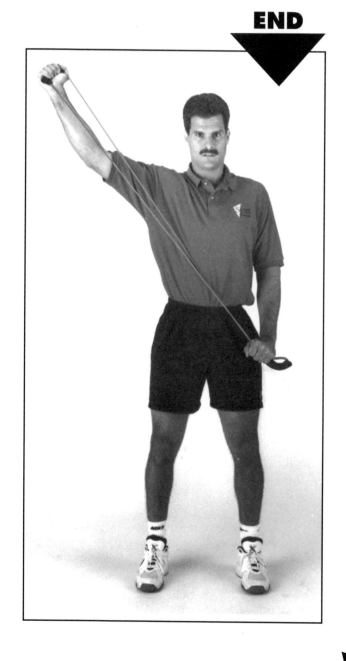

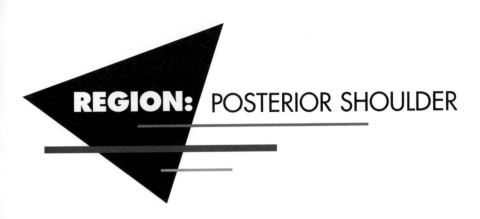

ULTRA TONER STANDING REVERSE FLYE

(Posterior Deltoid)

A. Stand in a square stance, soften knees, keep hips back, pelvis tilted slightly anterior and lumbar spine neutral. Grasp both handles and extend arms straight out from shoulders in a thumbs up position.

B. With firm wrists and a slight bend in elbows, pull back until shoulder blades are squeezed together.

C. Hands end parallel to and slightly behind shoulders in a thumbs up position. Mid-point pad should be in contact with upper chest.

D. Keep the chest up, rib cage lifted, bellybutton drawn toward spine and the lumbar spine in its neutral curvature.

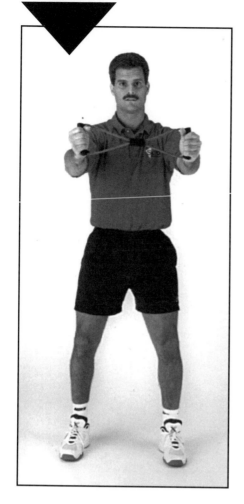

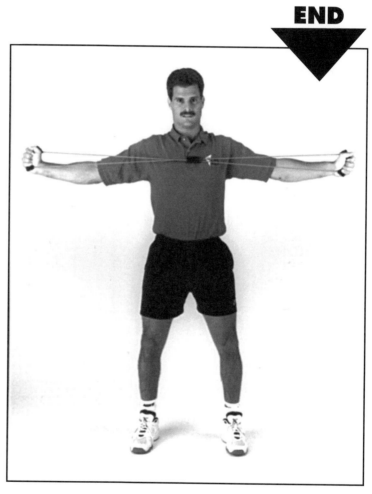

THE COMPLETE GUIDE TO **RUBBERIZED RESISTANCE EXERCISES** 261

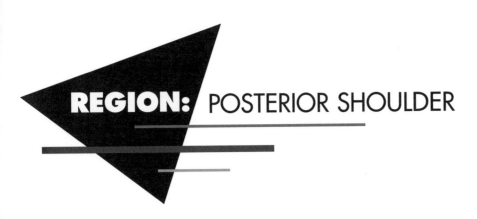

REGION: POSTERIOR SHOULDER

ULTRA TONER BENT OVER SINGLE ARM REVERSE FLYE

(Posterior Deltoid)

A. Position feet slightly wider than shoulder width, bend over so chest is approximately parallel to floor, and assume a half-squat position.

B. Grasp a handle with your exercising hand. With your other hand, grasp mid-point pad, or other handle, and rest it just above your opposite side knee.

C. With firm wrist, pull up and out across body. The hand will progress to a palm down position as arm fully extends out from shoulder. Shoulders must stay square.

D. Keep the chest up, rib cage lifted, bellybutton drawn toward spine and the lumbar spine in its neutral curvature.

E. Switch hand positions and repeat equal amounts of repetitions with other hand.

START

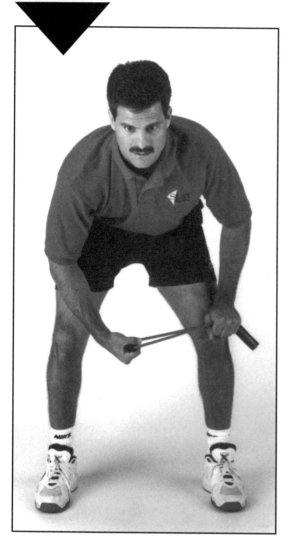

END

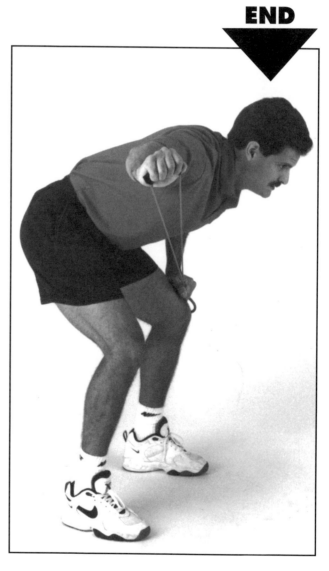

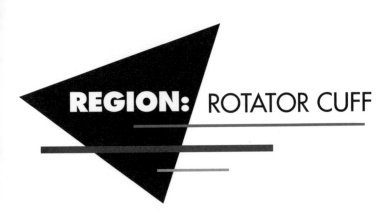

REGION: ROTATOR CUFF

ULTRA TONER STANDING EXTERNAL SHOULDER ROTATION

(External Rotators)

▼ **Position of shoulder joint - 0° Abduction (neutral position)**

A. Stand in a square or staggered stance. Soften knees, keep hips back, pelvis tilted slightly anterior and lumbar spine neutral.

B. Grasp handles with thumbs up and elbows flexed 90° directly under shoulders (neutral position). With firm wrists, gradually rotate shoulder outward by pulling away from body, performing a semicircular motion with lower arms.

C. Finish with thumbs pointing upward, elbows directly under shoulders externally rotated through their full range of motion.

D. Keep the chest up, rib cage lifted, bellybutton drawn toward spine and the lumbar spine in its neutral curvature.

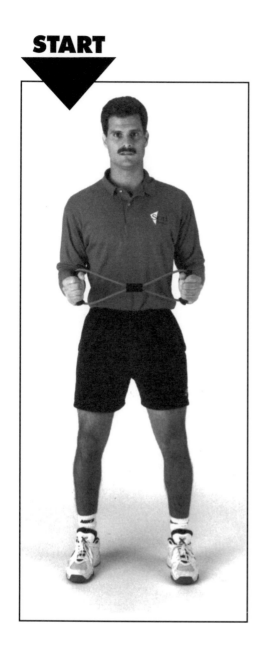

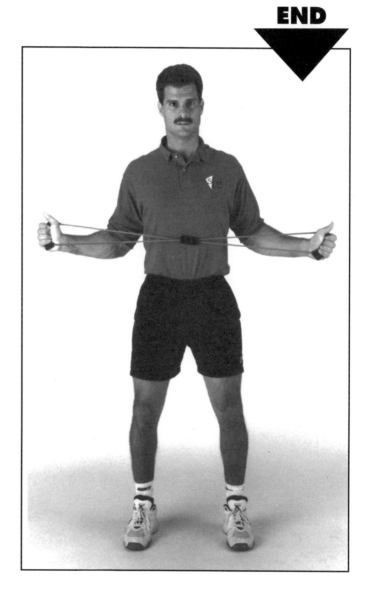

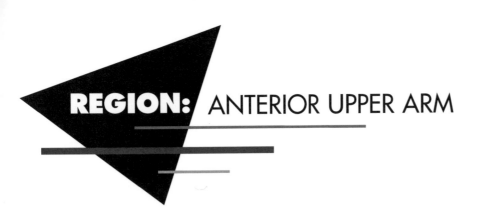

ULTRA TONER STANDING SINGLE ARM CURL

(Biceps)

▼ **Position of shoulder joint - Neutral**

A. Stand and place one foot into one end of Ultra Toner so handle rests under arch. Soften knees, keep hips back, pelvis tilted slightly anterior and lumbar spine neutral.

B. Grasp other handle with your same side hand and straighten arm directly under shoulder with thumb pointing forward.

C. Bend elbow and gradually supinate forearm so palm faces ceiling at hip level.

D. Continue bending elbow until fist faces ceiling. Palm of hand ends facing front portion of shoulder with thumb pointing out and away from side of body. Finish with elbow directly under shoulder.

E. Keep the chest up, rib cage lifted, bellybutton drawn toward spine and the lumbar spine in its neutral curvature.

F. Place handle under other foot and repeat equal amounts of repetitions with other hand.

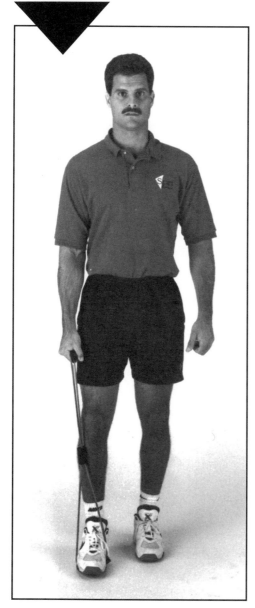

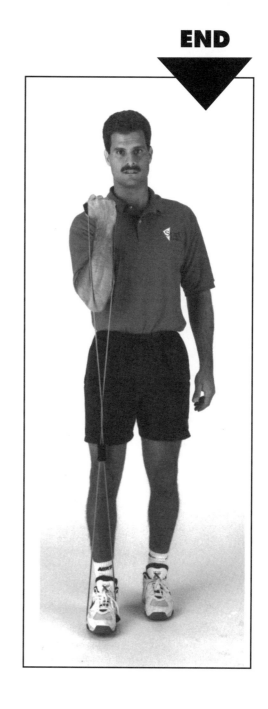

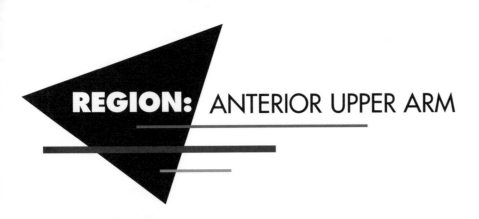

REGION: ANTERIOR UPPER ARM

ULTRA TONER SEATED SINGLE ARM CURL
(Biceps)

▼ **Position of shoulder joint - Frontal**

A. Sit and place one foot into one end of Ultra Toner so handle rests under arch and grasp other handle with your same side hand.

B. Extend leg fully, keeping hand and foot in a straight line with shoulder. Place other hand on opposite bent knee.

C. Sit upright and position exercising hand above same side knee in a thumb up position.

D. Bend elbow and gradually supinate forearm so palm faces ceiling while flexing shoulder slightly. Curl fully, ending with palm facing front of shoulder. Shoulder ends flexed approximately 80° with elbow slightly under shoulder.

E. Keep the chest up, rib cage lifted, bellybutton drawn toward spine and the lumbar spine in its neutral curvature.

F. Place handle under other foot and repeat equal amounts of repetitions with other hand.

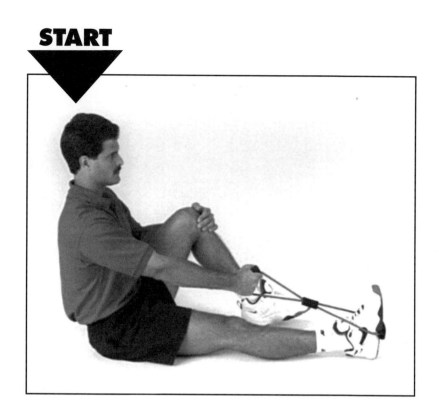

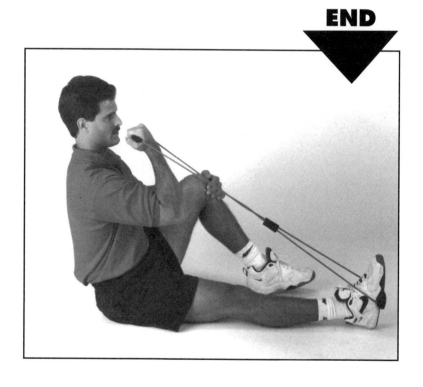

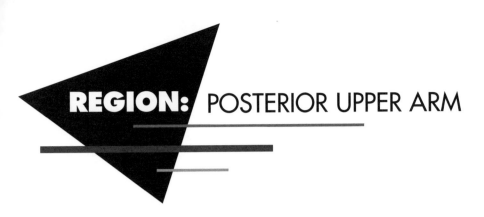

REGION: POSTERIOR UPPER ARM

ULTRA TONER STANDING SINGLE ARM PRESS DOWN

(Triceps)

▼ **Position of shoulder joint - Neutral**

A. Assume a square stance slightly wider than shoulder width and soften knees. Keep hips back, pelvis tilted slightly anterior and lumbar spine neutral.

B. Grasp mid-point pad or a handle with your non-exercising hand and extend arm out from and above same side shoulder. Palm should face forward.

C. Grasp other handle with your exercising hand and place your palm across from upper chest on opposite side of body.

D. With a firm wrist, press down and across body straightening arm fully. End with palm facing outer thigh and hand directly under shoulder.

E. Keep the chest up, rib cage lifted, bellybutton drawn toward spine and the lumbar spine in its neutral curvature.

F. Switch arm positions and repeat equal amounts of repetitions with other hand.

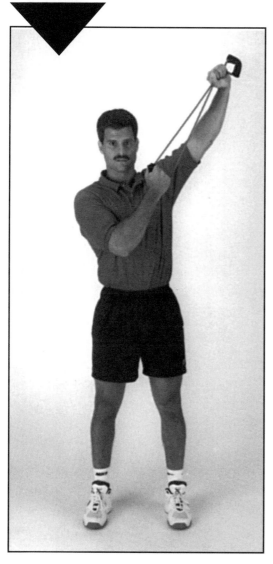

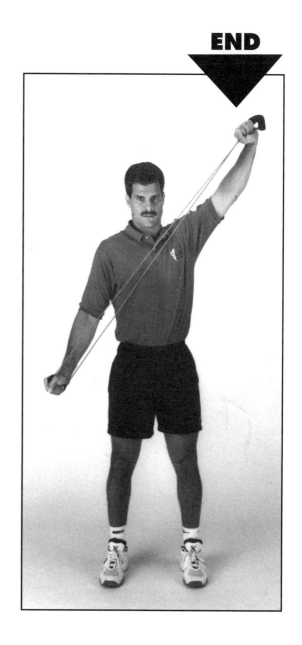

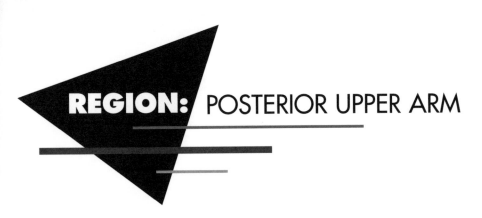

REGION: POSTERIOR UPPER ARM

ULTRA TONER STANDING BEHIND NECK PRESS OUT

(Triceps)

▼ **Position of shoulder joint - Frontal**

A. Assume a square stance slightly wider than shoulder width and soften knees. Keep hips back, pelvis tilted slightly anterior and lumbar spine neutral.

B. Position mid-point pad of Ultra Toner behind neck. Bend arms and position elbows directly to sides of shoulders with upper arms parallel to floor. Palms should face each other.

C. With firm wrists, press out straightening arms fully. End with palms facing up and hands in direct line with shoulders.

D. Keep the chest up, rib cage lifted, bellybutton drawn toward spine and the lumbar spine in its neutral curvature.

END

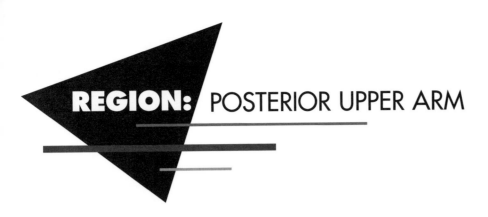

REGION: POSTERIOR UPPER ARM

ULTRA TONER STANDING SINGLE ARM BEHIND BACK PRESS UP

(Triceps)

▼ **Position of shoulder joint - Frontal**

A. Assume a square stance slightly wider than shoulder width and soften knees. Keep hips back, pelvis tilted slightly anterior and lumbar spine neutral.

B. Grasp a handle with your non-exercising hand, bend arm and place behind back with backside of hand against waistline.

C. Reach around back and grasp other handle with your exercising hand. Raise elbow directly above shoulder with thumb pointing down.

D. With firm wrist, press up gradually, pronating forearm and straightening arm fully. End with hand directly over shoulder and palm facing forward with knuckles facing ceiling.

E. Keep the chest up, rib cage lifted, bellybutton drawn toward spine and the lumbar spine in its neutral curvature.

F. Switch arm positions and repeat equal amounts of repetitions with other hand.

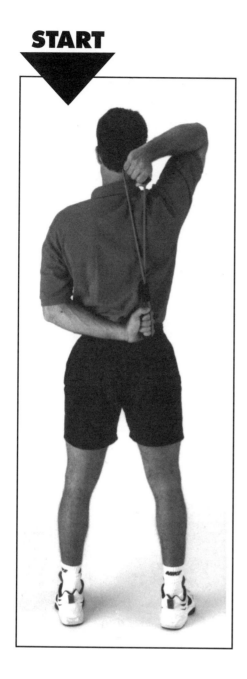

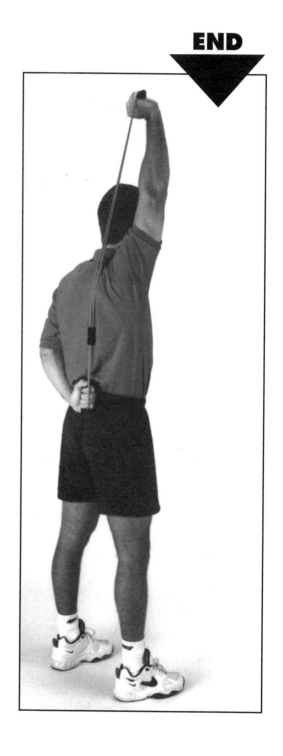

ULTRA TONER SEATED FULL/TERMINAL KNEE EXTENSION

(Quadriceps)

A. Place mid-point pad under arch of non-exercising foot and position open loop just above exercising ankle.

B. Sit upright on front edge of chair or bench and hold onto armrests or underside. Place a pad or rolled up towel under knees for extra comfort if desired.

C. Place both feet on floor directly under knees.

D. 1. FULL KNEE EXTENSION - Extend knee of exercising leg. Lift up to height of knee until the quadricep is fully contracted.

   2. TERMINAL KNEE EXTENSION - Move leg forward, placing heel on floor, to a one-third flexed knee position. Extend knee of exercising leg. Lift up to height of knee until the quadricep is fully contracted.

E. Keep the chest up, rib cage lifted, bellybutton drawn toward spine and the lumbar spine in its neutral curvature.

F. Switch foot positions and repeat equal amounts of repetitions with other leg.

START
(D1)

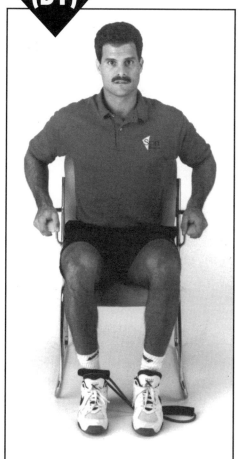

START
(D2)

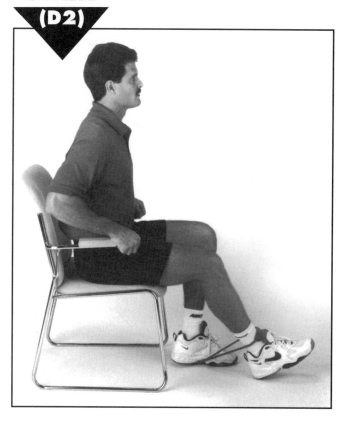

END

(D1 & D2)

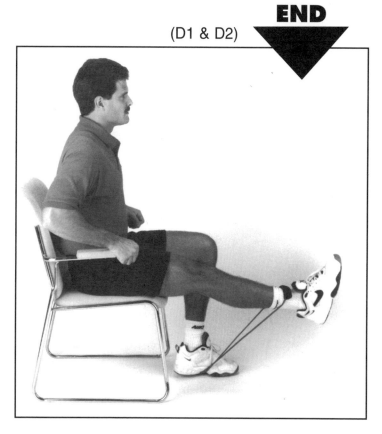

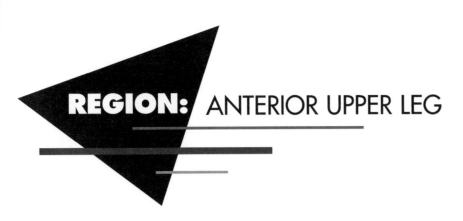

ULTRA TONER SEATED STRAIGHT LEG HIP FLEXION/BENT LEG KNEE EXTENSION

(Hip Flexors/Quadriceps)

▼ **Position - Elbow Supported**

A. Place Ultra Toner wrap under arch of non-exercising foot and position open loop just above exercising ankle.

B. Lie back supporting upper body on elbows.

C. 1. HIP FLEXION - Extend exercising leg fully and bend non-exercising leg. Keep ankle neutral and raise leg upward to approximately 45°- 60° of hip flexion.

2. KNEE EXTENSION - Bend both legs. Extend knee of exercising leg. Lift up to height of knee until quadricep is fully contracted.

D. Keep the chest up, rib cage lifted, bellybutton drawn toward spine and the lumbar spine in its neutral curvature.

E. Switch foot positions and repeat equal amounts of repetitions with other leg.

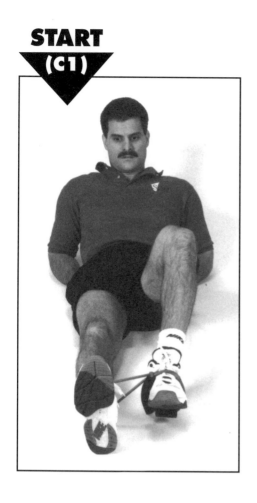

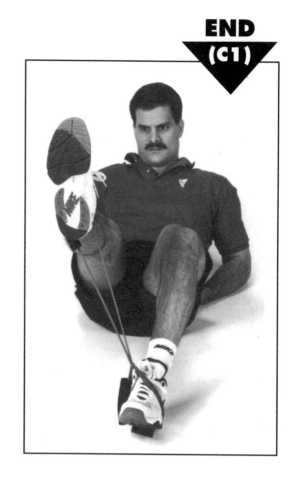

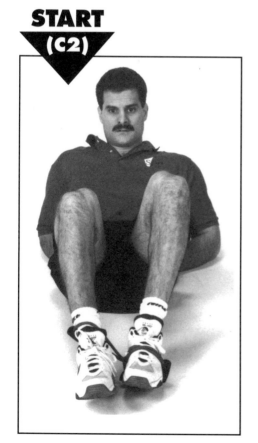

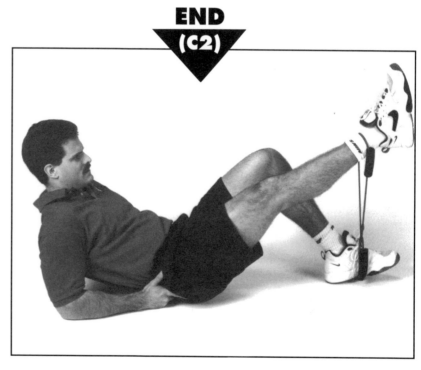

ULTRA TONER STANDING STRAIGHT LEG HIP FLEXION

(Hip Flexors/Rectus Femoris of Quadricep)

A. Place mid-point pad under arch of non-exercising foot and position open loop just above exercising ankle.

B. Place hands on hips or hold onto an object at the side of the body at waist height if stabilization is too demanding.

C. Keep foot of non-exercising leg on floor, knee slightly bent and non-exercising hip stationary. Hips and shoulders must remain square throughout exercise.

D. Keep ankle neutral and raise upward to approximately 45-60° of hip flexion.

E. Keep the chest up, rib cage lifted, bellybutton drawn toward spine and the lumbar spine in its neutral curvature.

F. Switch foot positions and repeat equal amounts of repetitions with other leg.

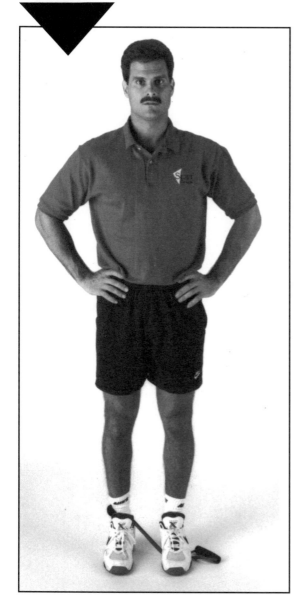

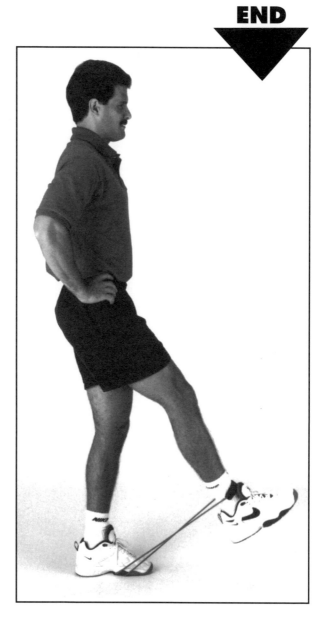

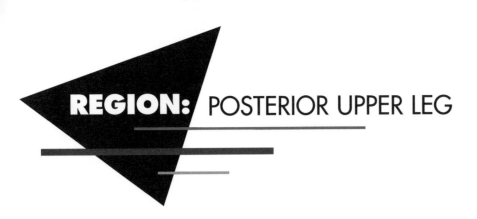

ULTRA TONER SEATED TERMINAL KNEE FLEXION

(Hamstrings)

A. Place Ultra Toner wrap just above non-exercising ankle and position open loop just above exercising ankle.

B. Sit upright on front edge of chair or bench, and hold onto armrests or underside. Place a pad or rolled up towel under knees for extra comfort if desired.

C. Move legs forward, placing heels of exercising leg on floor in a one-third flexed knee position. Keep non-exercising heel on floor, flex knee and curl buttocks until hamstring is fully contracted.

D. Keep the chest up, rib cage lifted, bellybutton drawn toward spine and the lumbar spine in its neutral curvature.

E. Switch foot positions and repeat equal amounts of repetitions with other leg.

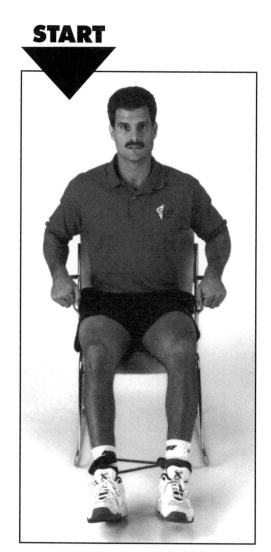

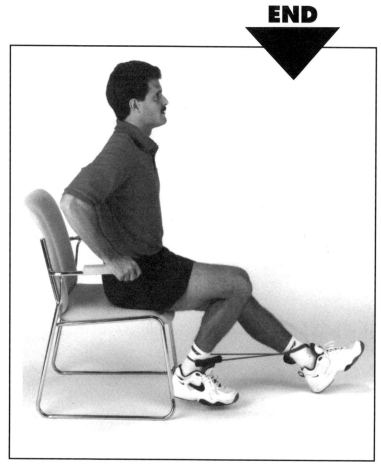

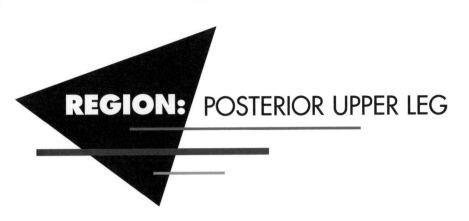

ULTRA TONER PRONE STRAIGHT LEG HIP EXTENSION

(Hamstrings/Gluteals)

▼ Position - Off Elevated Platform

A. Place Ultra Toner wrap just above non-exercising ankle and position open loop just above exercising ankle.

B. Lie on stomach and position hip bones comfortably over edge.

C. With toes of both feet on floor and legs extended, straighten arms overhead and grasp underside of bench or platform.

D. Pull toes of exercising foot toward shin to a neutral position.

E. Keep hip bones and chin in contact with bench or platform. The toes of the non-exercising foot should remain in contact with the floor.

F. Push exercising leg up and back, and gradually turn foot out slightly until gluteal is fully contracted. The exercise leg should end slightly out and away from midline of body.

G. Switch Ultra Toner wrap and repeat equal amounts of repetitions with other leg.

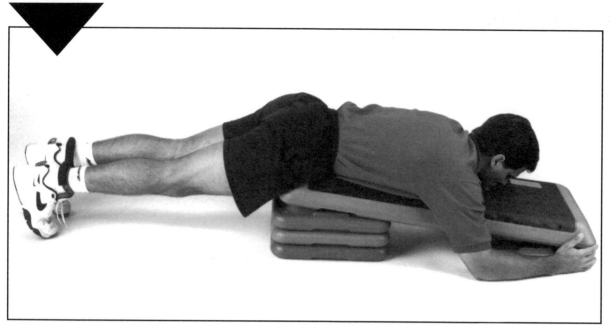

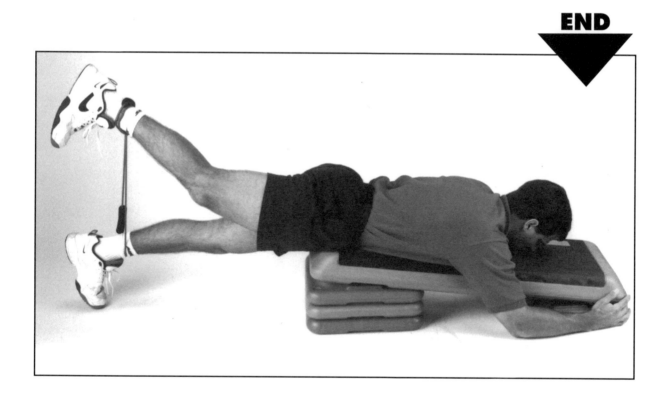

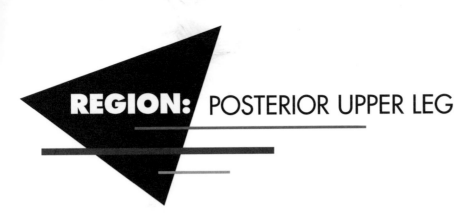

ULTRA TONER STANDING STRAIGHT LEG HIP-HYPEREXTENSION

(Hamstrings/Gluteals)

A. Place mid-point pad under arch of non-exercising foot and position open loop just above exercising ankle.

B. Stagger feet so foot of exercising leg is slightly behind foot of non-exercising leg. Pull toes of exercising foot toward shin to a neutral ankle position.

C. Place hands on hips or hold onto an object out in front of body at waist height if stabilization is too demanding.

D. Keep foot of non-exercising leg on floor, knee slightly bent and non-exercising hip stationary. Hips and shoulders must remain square throughout exercise.

E. Push exercising leg back and gradually turn foot out slightly until gluteal is fully contracted. The exercise leg should end slightly out and away from midline of body.

F. Keep the chest up, rib cage lifted, bellybutton drawn toward spine and the lumbar spine in its neutral curvature.

G. Switch foot positions and repeat equal amounts of repetitions with other leg.

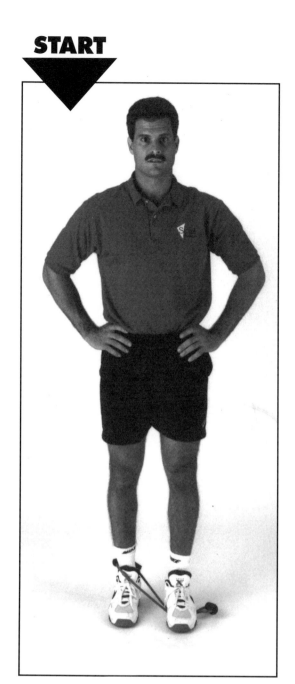

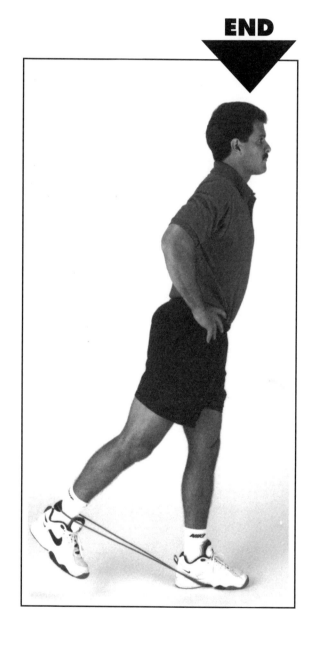

ULTRA TONER QUADRAPED MULE KICK

(Hamstrings/Gluteals)

A. Position body with all fours on the floor. Place one handle of Ultra Toner slightly above a knee. Place other handle under arch of opposite side foot. Support upper body on elbows and forearms.

B. Pull toes of exercising foot toward shin to a neutral ankle position.

C. Maintain natural arch in lower back, keep hips and shoulders square.

D. Push exercising leg up and back and gradually turn foot out slightly until gluteal is fully contracted. The exercise leg should end slightly out and away from midline of body.

E. Keep the chest up, rib cage lifted, bellybutton drawn toward spine and the lumbar spine in its neutral curvature.

F. Place handle slightly above other knee and repeat equal amounts of repetitions with other leg.

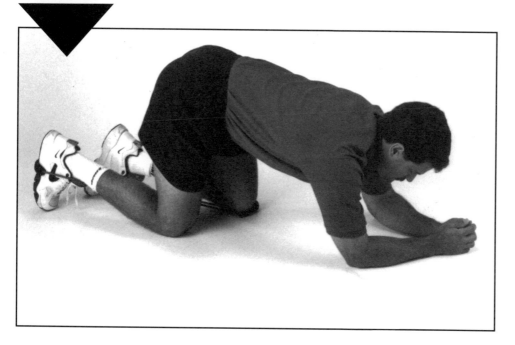

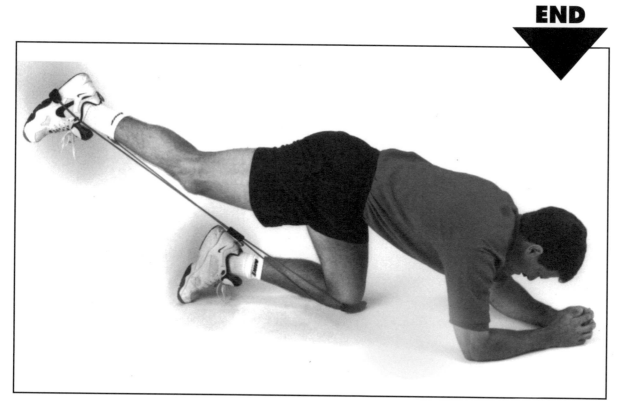

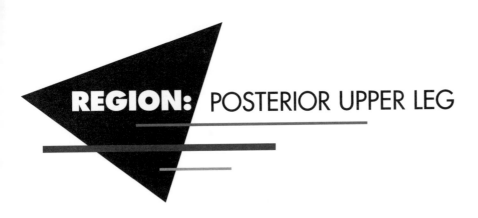

ULTRA TONER STANDING LEG CURL

(Hamstrings)

A. Place mid-point pad under arch of non-exercising foot and position open loop just above exercising ankle.

B. Stagger feet so foot of exercising leg is slightly behind foot of non-exercising leg. Pull toes of exercising foot toward shin to a neutral ankle position.

C. Place hands on hips or hold onto an object out in front of body at waist height if stabilization is too demanding.

D. Keep foot of non-exercising leg on floor, knee slightly bent, and non-exercising hip stationary. Hips and shoulders must remain square throughout exercise.

E. Flex knee and curl leg toward buttocks until hamstring is fully contracted.

F. Keep the chest up, rib cage lifted, bellybutton drawn toward spine and the lumbar spine in its neutral curvature.

G. Switch foot positions and repeat equal amounts of repetitions with other leg.

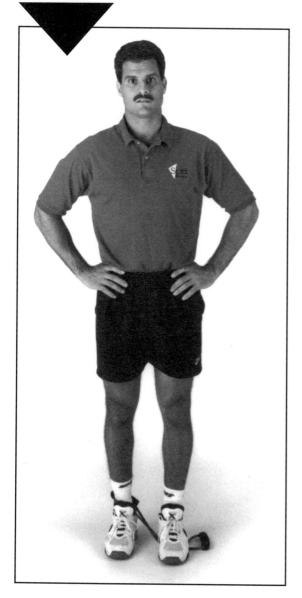

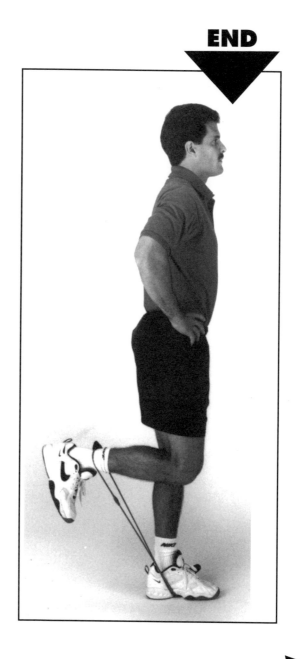

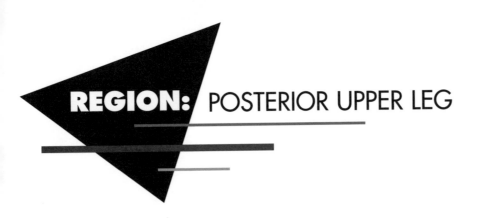

ULTRA TONER PRONE LEG CURL
(Hamstrings)

A. Place Ultra Toner around non-exercising foot arch and position open loop just above exercising ankle.

B. Lie on stomach, place back of hands under chin and extend both legs. Place a pad or rolled up towel under knee of exercising leg for extra comfort if desired.

C. Pull toes of exercising foot toward shin to a neutral ankle position.

D. Keep hip bones in contact with floor, flex knee and curl leg toward buttocks until hamstring is fully contracted.

E. Switch Ultra Toner wrap and repeat equal amounts of repetitions with other leg.

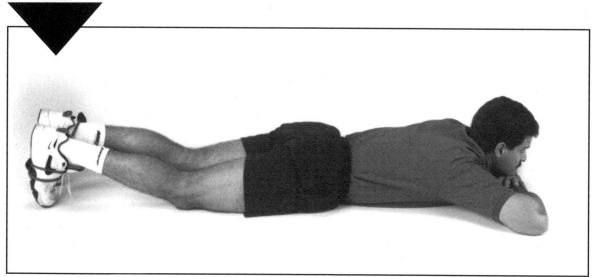

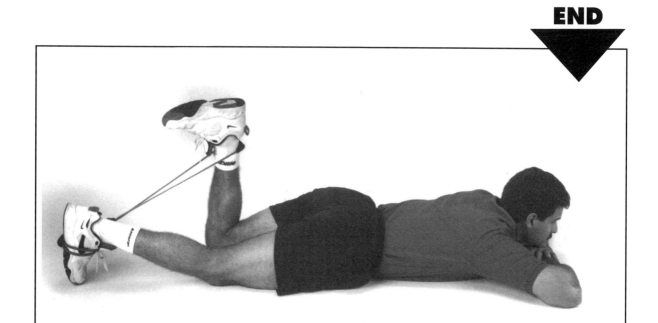

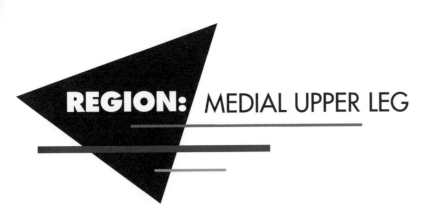

ULTRA TONER SEATED STRAIGHT LEG HIP ADDUCTION

(Adductors/Hip Internal Rotators)

▼ Position - Elbow or Hand Supported

A. From a seated position, place one open loop of Ultra Toner around exercising lower leg at calf height. If needed, place open loop higher toward knees to lessen resistance and decrease stress upon knee ligaments.

B. Have partner hold other end of Ultra Toner taut or use attachable door strap and anchor at ankle height. Partner or attachment is positioned outside exercising leg.

C. With exercising leg fully abducted, lie back supporting upper body on elbows or with hands. The exercising leg should be straightened with hip externally rotated so toes point outward.

D. Keep leg straight, pull up and in toward bent knee while gradually rotating hip inward. End knee to knee, toes inward, and adductors fully contracted.

E. Keep the chest up, rib cage lifted, bellybutton drawn toward spine and the lumbar spine in its neutral curvature.

F. Place Ultra Toner around other lower leg and repeat equal amounts of repetitions.

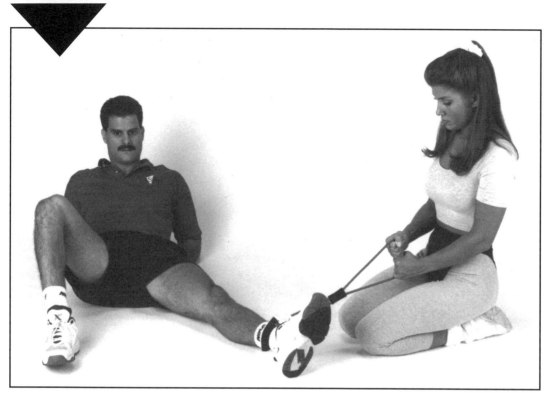

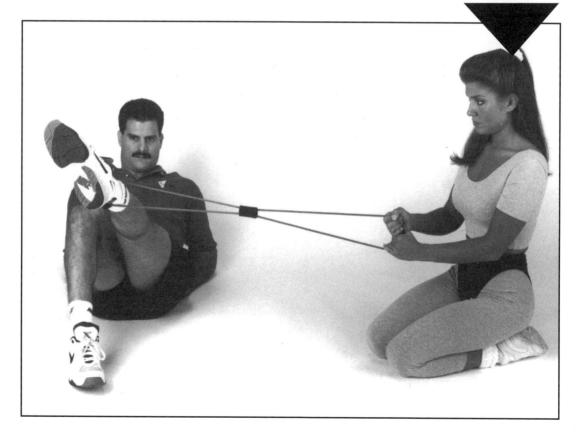

THE COMPLETE GUIDE TO **RUBBERIZED RESISTANCE EXERCISES** 295

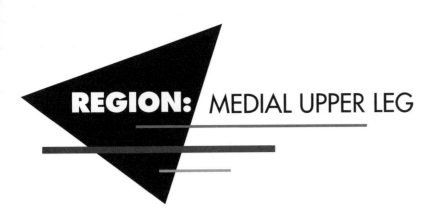

ULTRA TONER STANDING STRAIGHT/BENT LEG HIP ADDUCTION

(Adduction/Hip Internal Rotators)

A. From a standing position, place one open loop of Ultra Toner around exercising lower leg at calf height. If needed, place open loop higher toward knees to lessen resistance and decrease stress upon knee ligaments.

B. Have partner hold other end of Ultra Toner taut or use attachable door strap and anchor at mid-calf height. Partner or attachment is positioned outside exercising leg.

C. Keep foot of non-exercising leg on floor, knee slightly bent and non-exercising hip stationary with gluteals, hamstrings, and quadriceps contracted. Hips and shoulders must remain square throughout exercise.

D. With exercising leg fully abducted, place hands on hips or hold onto an object at side of body at waist height if stabilization is too demanding.

E. STRAIGHT LEG - Keep leg straight, lead with heel, pull forward and inward until adductors are fully contracted. End slightly in front of non-exercising foot. Do not allow the hip and knee of non-exercising leg to rotate.

BENT LEG - Lead with knee, drive it up and inward until adductors are fully contracted. End with heel in contact with inside of non-exercising knee.

F. Keep the chest up, rib cage lifted, bellybutton drawn toward spine and the lumbar spine in its neutral curvature.

G. Place Ultra Toner around other lower leg and repeat equal amounts of repetitions.

START

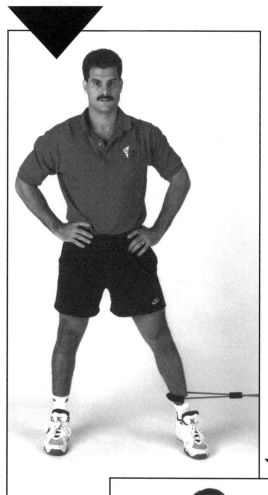

END

STRAIGHT LEG

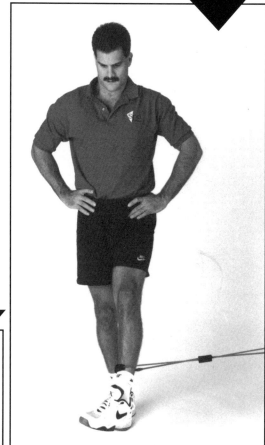

END

BENT LEG

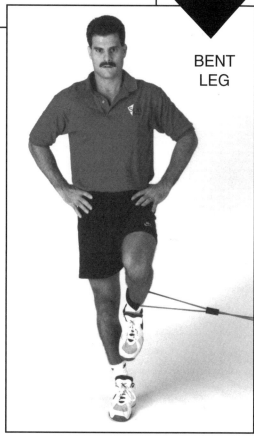

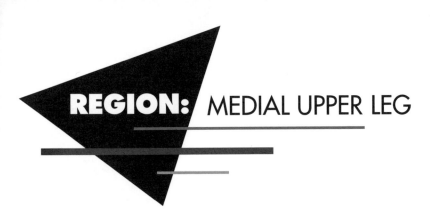

ULTRA TONER SIDE LYING STRAIGHT LEG HIP ADDUCTION

(Adductors)

A. From a seated position, bend non-exercising leg fully so heel is parallel to opposite knee. Place mid-point pad of Ultra Toner under arch of foot and point toes forward.

B. Place other end of Ultra Toner at mid-calf height of exercising leg and straighten.

C. Lie on side and roll onto hip of exercising leg. Rotate hip outward so toes point away from body.

D. Bend arm and support body weight on elbow. Place other hand across body on floor to stabilize pelvis.

E. Keep leg straight, lead with heel and pull up and in toward bent knee until adductors are fully contracted. End with knees parallel to one another.

F. Keep the chest up, rib cage lifted, bellybutton drawn toward spine and the lumbar spine in its neutral curvature.

G. Roll onto other side, switch foot positions and repeat equal amounts of repetitions with other leg.

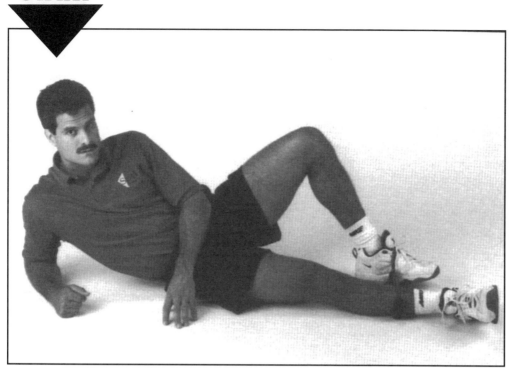

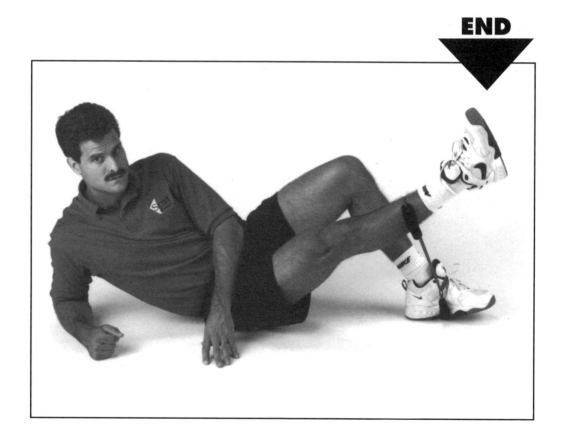

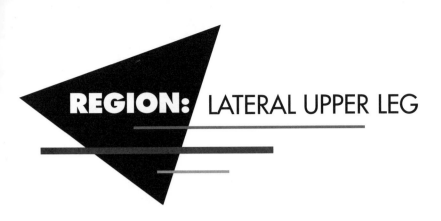

ULTRA TONER STANDING STRAIGHT LEG HIP ABDUCTION

(Abductors)

A. Place mid-point pad under arch of non-exercising foot and position open loop just above exercising ankle.

B. Place hands on hips or hold onto an object at side of body at waist height if stabilization is too demanding.

C. Rotate hip of exercising leg inward. Keep leg straight, lead with heel and push outward as far as possible. The opposite hip and shoulders must remain stationary.

D. Keep the chest up, rib cage lifted, bellybutton drawn toward spine and the lumbar spine in its neutral curvature.

E. Switch foot positions and repeat equal amounts of repetitions with other leg.

START

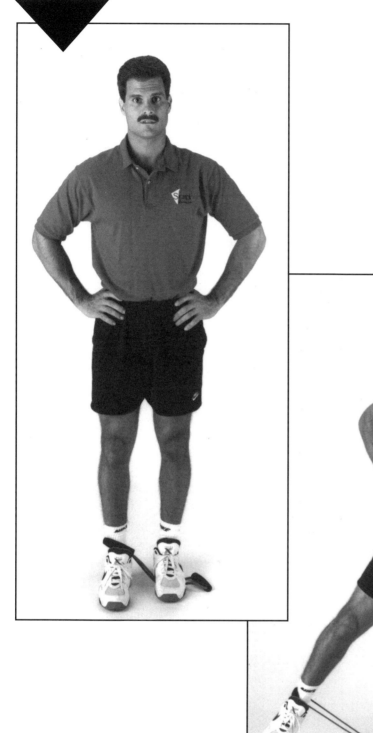

END

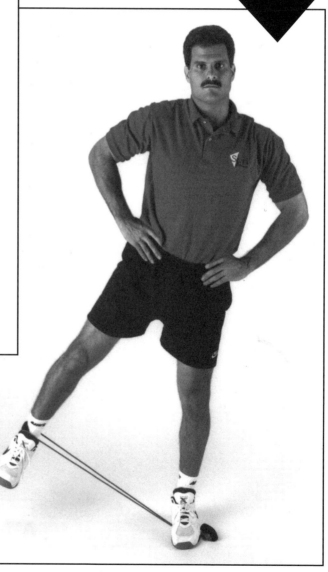

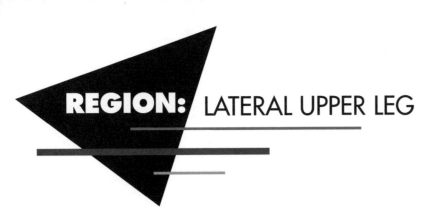

ULTRA TONER SIDE LYING STRAIGHT LEG HIP ABDUCTION

(Abductors)

A. Place Ultra Toner wrap just above non-exercising ankle and position open loop just above exercising ankle.

B. Lie on side and roll onto hip of non-exercising leg.

C. Bend arm that rests on floor overhead and place head on shoulder. Place other hand across body on floor to stabilize pelvis.

D. Extend both legs fully, lead with heel and push upward as high as possible. The opposite hip must remain stationary.

E. Keep the chest up, rib cage lifted, bellybutton drawn toward spine and the lumbar spine in its neutral curvature.

F. Roll onto other side, switch Ultra Toner wrap and repeat equal amounts of repetitions with other leg.

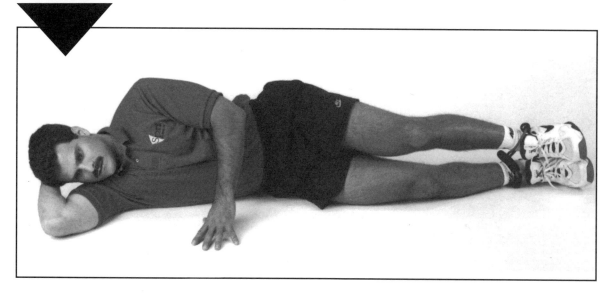

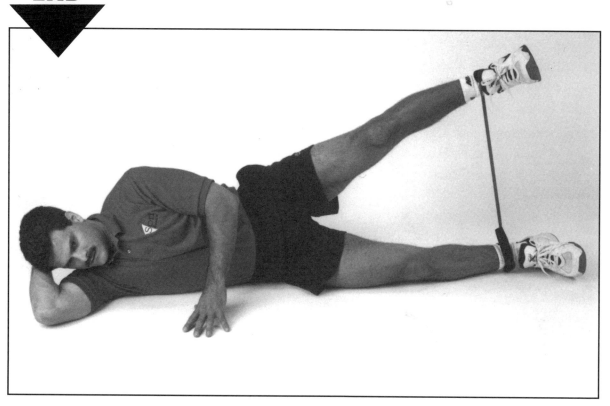

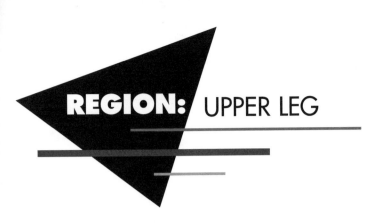

ULTRA TONER REVERSE BENT TRAIL LEG LUNGE

(Quadriceps/Hamstrings/Gluteals)

A. Stand in a narrow staggered lunge position. Place mid-point pad of Ultra Toner under arch of front foot.

B. Grasp handles and extend arms straight down from shoulders.

C. Take a drop step with other leg and land behind or on ball of foot. Bend knees and descend to form a 90° angle with upper and lower portion of each leg. The kneecap of lead leg should be over the mid-foot. Keep heel down and weight distributed evenly through front foot. Heel of trail leg is up off floor, knee slightly behind hip and ball of foot is in contact with floor.

D. Keep head over hips and eyes focused directly forward. Keep the chest expanded, rib cage lifted, shoulder blades squeezed together, bellybutton drawn toward spine and the lumbar spine in its neutral curvature.

E. STATIONARY - Keep feet in this position, straighten both lead and trail legs simultaneously. Stand tall through ball of trail leg foot and squeeze gluteal muscles.

DYNAMIC - Return to start position and repeat drop step (point C).

F. Switch foot positions and repeat equal amounts of repetitions with other leg.

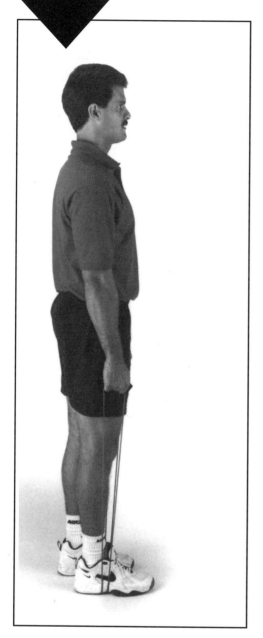

END

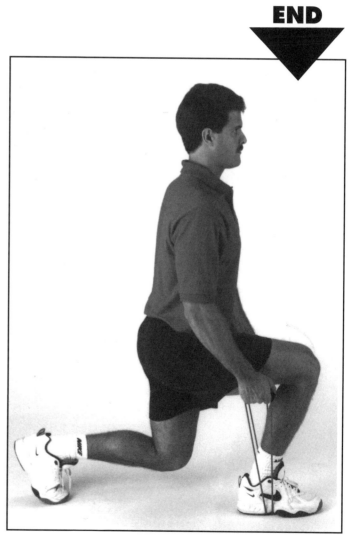

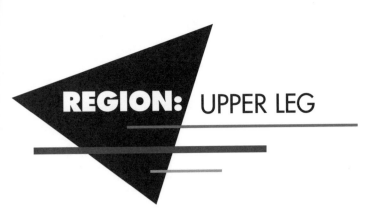

REGION: UPPER LEG

ULTRA TONER BACK LYING SINGLE LEG PRESS

(Quadriceps/Hamstrings/Gluteals)

A. Lie on back, bend non-exercising leg fully so heel is slightly forward of knee with foot flat. Grasp handles of Ultra Toner and place mid-point pad under arch of exercising foot. Keep elbows in contact with floor.

B. Bring knee of exercising leg back over hip and pull toes toward shin to a neutral ankle position.

C. Keep kneecap in alignment with foot and straighten leg fully, contracting upper leg musculature.

D. Switch foot positions and repeat equal amounts of repetitions with other leg.

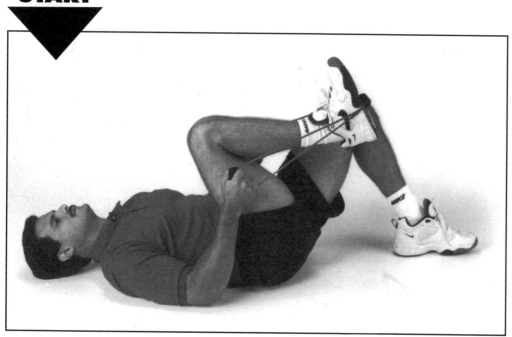

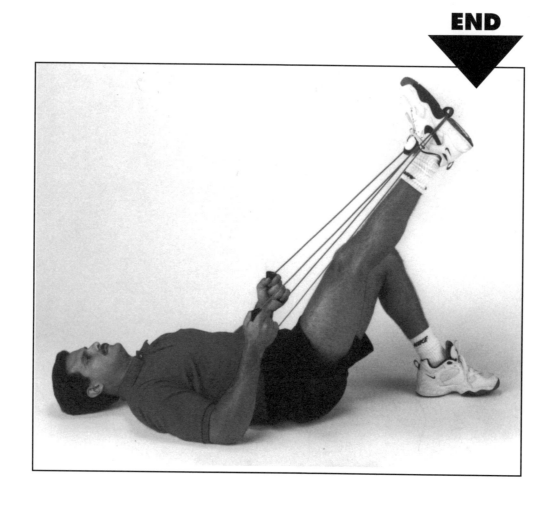

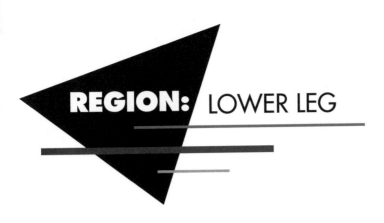

ULTRA TONER SEATED ANKLE PLANTAR FLEXION

(Ankle Plantar Flexors)

A. Sit on floor with exercising leg straight and non-exercising leg fully bent with heel slightly forward of knee with foot flat.

B. Grasp handles of Ultra Toner and place mid-point pad around ball of straight leg foot.

C. Raise heel off floor, keep thigh stationary, and press toes downward against mid-point pad as far as possible (plantar flexion).

D. Contraction should be felt in back of lower leg.

E. Keep the chest up, rib cage lifted, bellybutton drawn toward spine and the lumbar spine in its neutral curvature.

F. Switch foot positions and repeat equal amounts of repetitions with other leg.

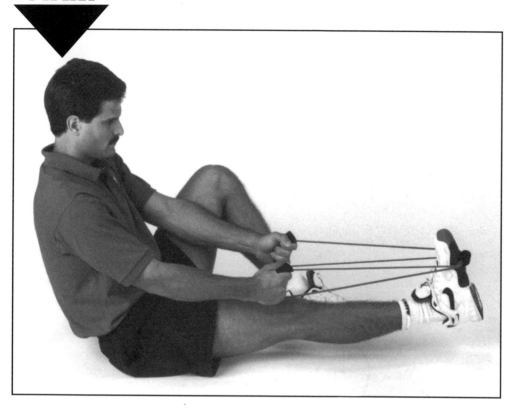

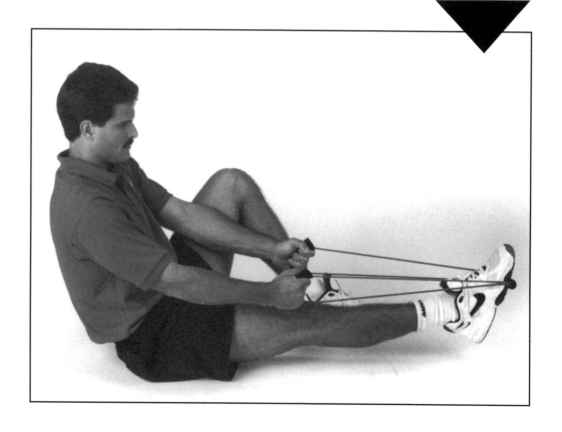

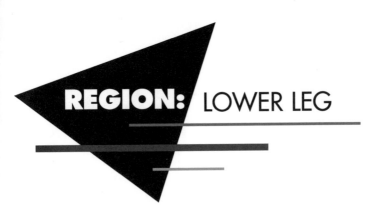

ULTRA TONER SEATED ANKLE EVERSION (Dual)

(Ankle Evertors)

A. Sit on floor and place open loops of Ultra Toner around forefoot of both feet. Place hands under shoulders.

B. Separate legs as far as needed for proper tension and point toes inward.

C. Keep thighs stationary and push little toes outward as far as possible (eversion).

D. Contraction should be felt in outer portion of ankle and lower leg.

E. Keep the chest up, rib cage lifted, bellybutton drawn toward spine and the lumbar spine in its neutral curvature.

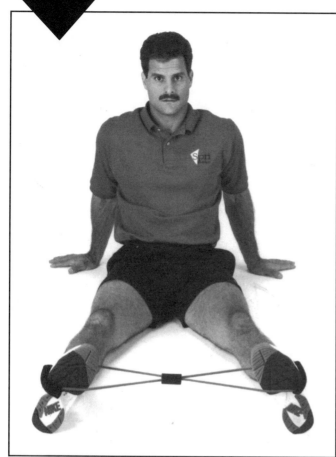

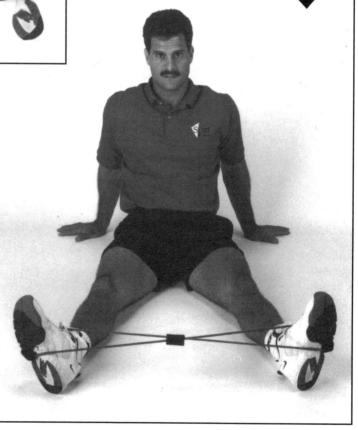

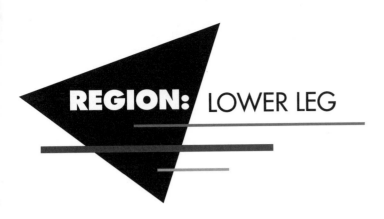

ULTRA TONER SEATED ANKLE INVERSION
(Ankle Invertors)

A. Sit on bench or elevated platform with ankles just over edge when using partner. Sit on floor and place pad or rolled up towel under calf of exercising leg if using attachable doorstop.

B. Place one open loop of Ultra Toner around exercising forefoot. Have partner hold other end of Ultra Toner taut or use attachable doorstrap and anchor at ankle height. Partner should place hand on exercising lower leg to stabilize hip. Partner or attachment is positioned outside exercising leg.

C. Rotate foot of exercising leg outward (eversion). Keep thigh stationary and pull big toe inward as far as possible (inversion).

D. Contraction should be felt in inner portion of ankle and lower leg.

E. Keep the chest up, rib cage lifted, bellybutton drawn toward spine and the lumbar spine in its neutral curvature.

F. Place Ultra Toner around other forefoot and repeat equal amounts of repetitions with other leg.

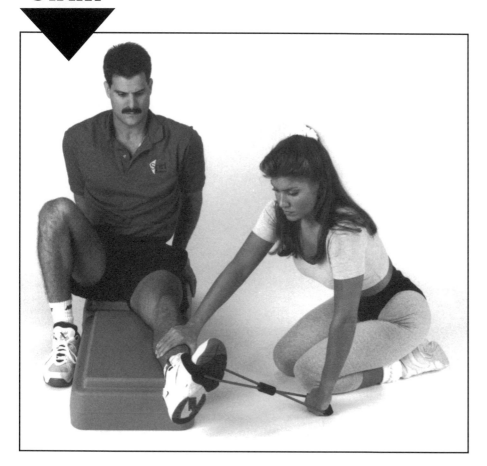

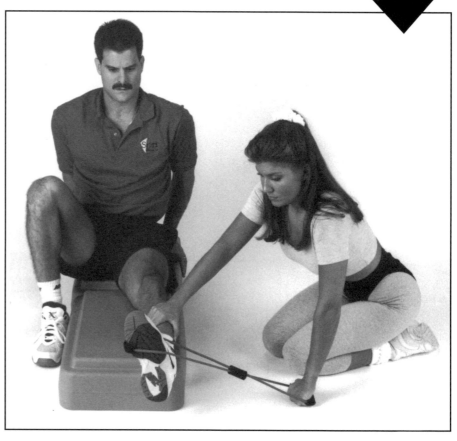

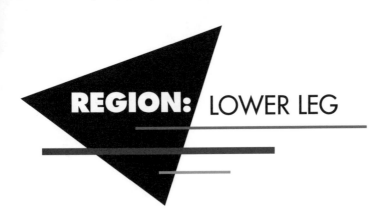

ULTRA TONER SEATED ANKLE DORSI FLEXION

(Ankle Dorsi Flexors)

A. Sit on bench or elevated platform with one ankle just over edge or sit on floor and place pad or rolled up towel under calf. Place hands behind body on floor or platform, bend other leg and place foot on floor, or heel on bench.

B. Bend knee slightly and place soft handle of Ultra Toner on top of forefoot. Have partner grasp mid-point pad, or handle, and hold taut. Partner is positioned in front of lower leg.

C. Keep thigh stationary and pull toes toward shin as far as possible (dorsi flexion).

D. Contraction should be felt in front lower leg.

E. Keep the chest up, rib cage lifted, bellybutton drawn toward spine and the lumbar spine in its neutral curvature.

F. Place Ultra Toner around other forefoot and repeat equal amounts of repetitions with other leg.

TECH TIPS
This exercise may be performed with both legs simultaneously using two Ultra Toners.

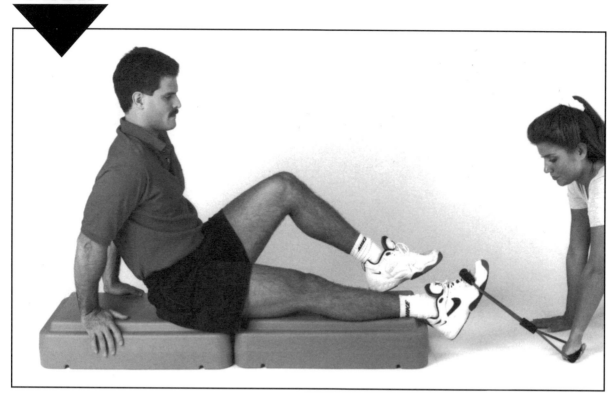

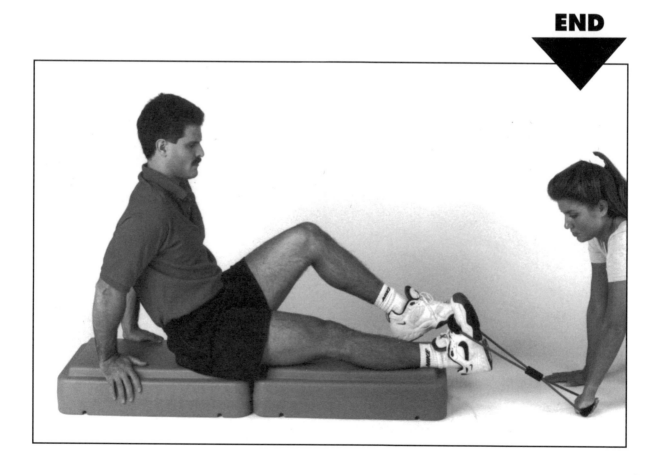

XERCISE BAND & XERING

XERCISE BAND™ RESISTANCE CHART

FLOOR EXERCISES DIMENSIONS	RESISTANCE
9" x 3/8" YELLOW	BEGINNER
9" x 5/8" GREEN	BEGINNER/INTERMEDIATE
12" x 3/4" RED	INTERMEDIATE/ADVANCED
9" x 1" BLUE	ADVANCED
FLOOR EXERCISES	RESISTANCE
12" x 1/2" GREEN	BEGINNER/INTERMEDIATE
9" x 3/4" RED	INTERMEDIATE/ADVANCED

XERING™ RESISTANCE CHART

COLOR	RESISTANCE
YELLOW	BEGINNER
GREEN	BEGINNER/INTERMEDIATE
RED	INTERMEDIATE/ADVANCED
BLUE	ADVANCED
BLACK	VERY ADVANCED

All exercises have been demonstrated with the Xercise Band but may be performed with the Xering.

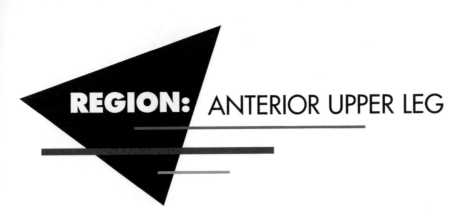

REGION: ANTERIOR UPPER LEG

XERCISE BAND SEATED FULL/TERMINAL KNEE EXTENSION

(Quadriceps)

A. Place Xercise Band around exercising lower leg just above ankle height and under non-exercising foot arch.

B. Sit upright on front edge of chair or bench and hold onto armrests or underside. Place a pad or rolled up towel under knees for extra comfort if desired.

C. Place both feet on floor directly under knees.

D. 1. Full Knee Extension - Extend knee of exercising leg. Lift up to height of knee until the quadricep is fully contracted.

2. Terminal Knee Extension - Move leg forward, placing heel on floor to a one-third flexed knee position. Extend knee of exercising leg. Lift up to height of knee until the quadricep is fully contracted.

E. Keep the chest up, rib cage lifted, bellybutton drawn toward spine and the lumbar spine in its neutral curvature.

F. Switch foot positions and repeat equal amounts of repetitions with other leg.

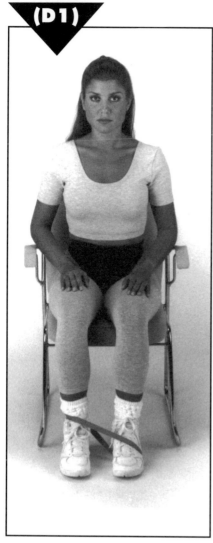

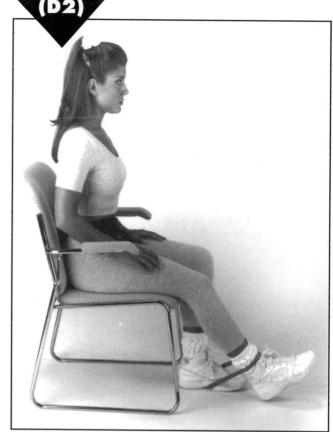

END

(D1 & D2)

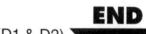

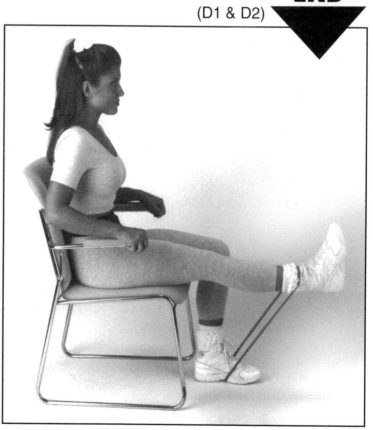

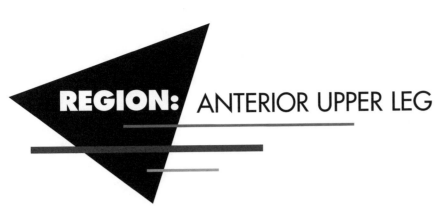

REGION: ANTERIOR UPPER LEG

XERCISE BAND SEATED STRAIGHT LEG HIP FLEXION/BENT LEG KNEE EXTENSION

(Hip Flexors/Quadriceps)

▼ Position - Elbow Supported

A. Place Xercise Band under arch of non-exercising foot and just above exercising ankle.

B. Lie back supporting upper body on elbows.

C. 1. Hip Flexion - Extend exercising leg fully and bend non-exercising leg. Keep ankle neutral and raise leg upward to approximately 45° - 60° of hip flexion.

   2. Knee Extension - Bend both legs. Extend knee of exercising leg. Lift up to height of knee until quadricep is fully contracted.

D. Keep the chest up, rib cage lifted, bellybutton drawn toward spine and the lumbar spine in its neutral curvature.

E. Switch foot positions and repeat equal amounts of repetitions with other leg.

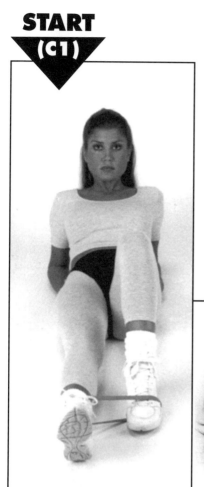

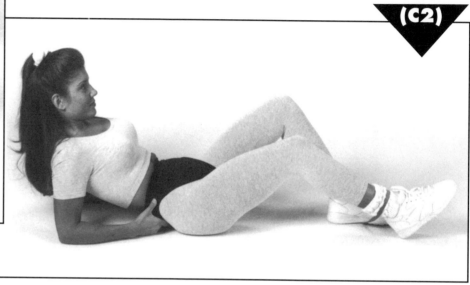

END
(C1 & C2)

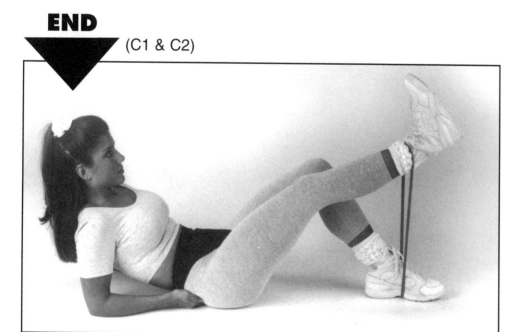

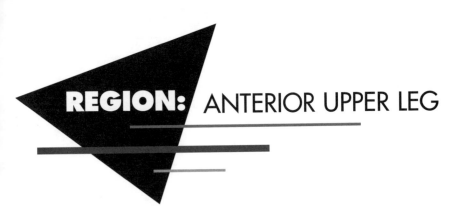

XERCISE BAND STANDING STRAIGHT LEG HIP FLEXION

(Hip Flexors/Rectus Femoris of Quadricep)

A. Place Xercise Band around both lower legs just above ankle height and assume a narrow stance.

B. Place hands on hips or hold onto an object at the side of the body at waist height if stabilization is too demanding.

C. Keep foot of non-exercising leg on floor, knee slightly bent and non-exercising hip stationary. Hips and shoulders must remain square throughout exercise.

D. Keep ankle neutral and raise upward to approximately 45° - 60° of hip flexion.

E. Keep the chest up, rib cage lifted, bellybutton drawn toward spine and the lumbar spine in its neutral curvature.

F. Repeat equal amounts of repetitions with other leg.

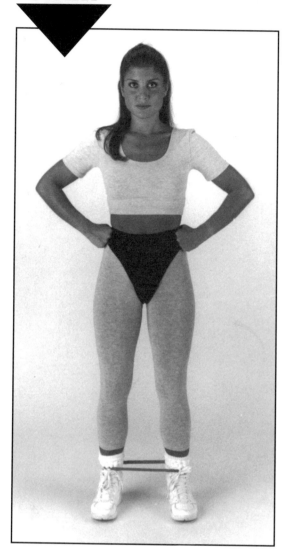

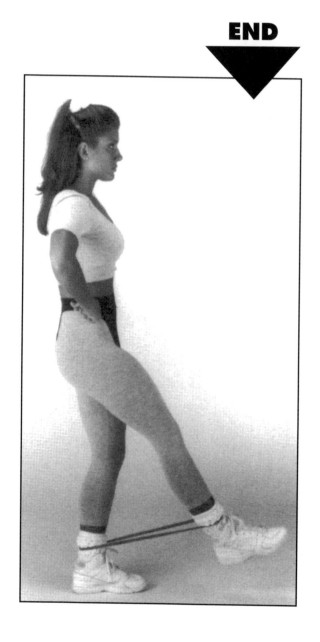

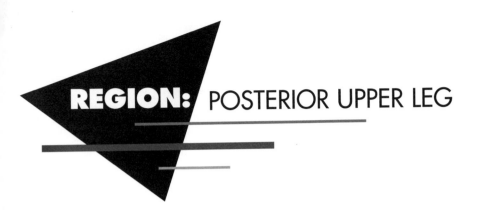

REGION: POSTERIOR UPPER LEG

XERCISE BAND SEATED TERMINAL KNEE FLEXION

(Hamstrings)

A. Place Xercise Band around exercising lower leg just above ankle height and around non-exercising foot arch.

B. Sit upright on front edge of chair or bench, and hold onto armrests or underside. Place a pad or rolled up towel under knees for extra comfort if desired.

C. Move legs forward placing heel of exercising leg on floor in a one-third flexed knee position. Keep non-exercising heel on floor, flex knee and curl toward buttocks until hamstring is fully contracted.

D. Keep the chest up, rib cage lifted, bellybutton drawn toward spine and the lumbar spine in its neutral curvature.

E. Switch foot positions and repeat equal amounts of repetitions with other leg.

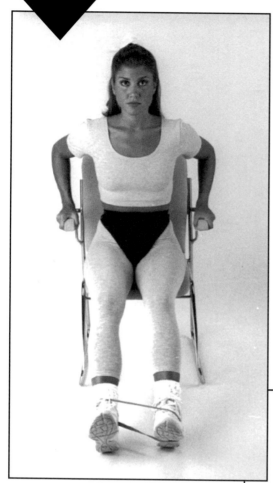

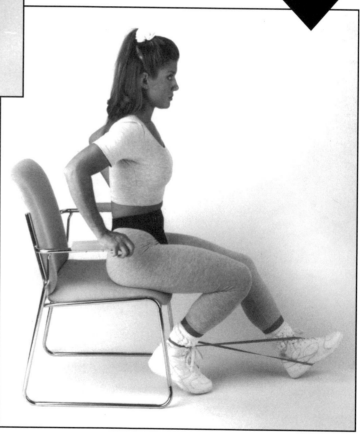

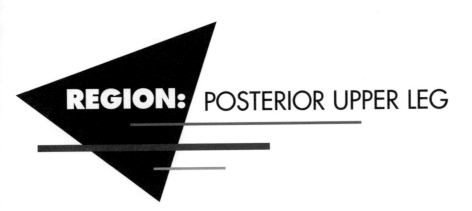

REGION: POSTERIOR UPPER LEG

XERCISE BAND PRONE STRAIGHT LEG HIP EXTENSION

(Hamstrings/Gluteals)

▼ Position - Off Elevated Platform

A. Place Xercise Band around both lower legs just above ankle height. Adjust bench or platform as high as necessary so lower legs fall below hip height.

B. Lie on stomach and position hip bones comfortably over edge.

C. With toes of both feet on floor, and legs extended, straighten arms overhead and grasp underside of bench or platform.

D. Pull toes of exercising foot toward shin to a neutral position.

E. Keep hip bones and chin in contact with bench or platform. The toes of the non-exercising foot should remain in contact with floor.

F. 1. Push exercising leg up and back and gradually turn foot out slightly until gluteal is fully contracted. The exercising leg should end slightly out and away from midline of body.

   2. For an advanced movement pattern, a leg curl may be added once hip is fully extended.

G. Repeat equal amounts of repetitions with other leg.

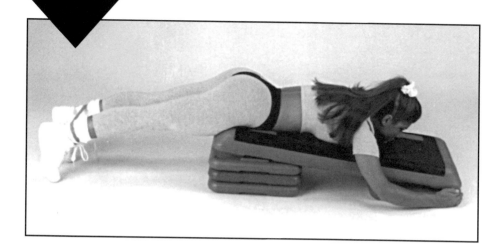

END (F1)

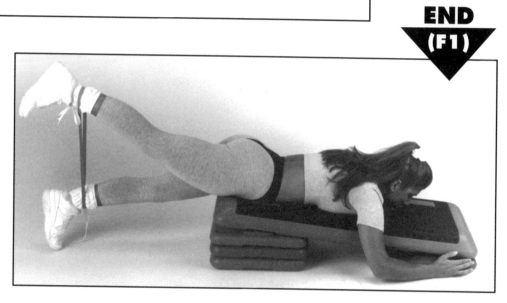

END (F2)

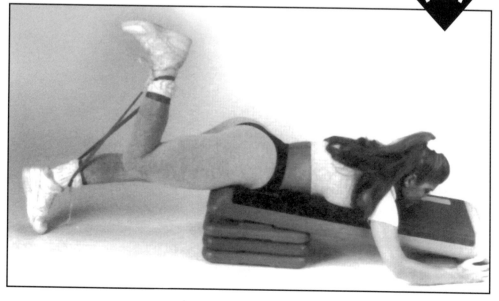

XERCISE BAND STANDING STRAIGHT LEG HIP-HYPEREXTENSION

(Hamstrings/Gluteals)

A. Place Xercise Band around both lower legs just above ankle height.

B. Stagger feet so foot of exercising leg is straight and slightly behind foot of non-exercising leg. Point toes of exercising leg down and keep them in contact with floor with heel up.

C. Place hands on hips or hold onto an object out in front of body at waist height if stabilization is too demanding.

D. Keep foot of non-exercising leg on floor, knee slightly bent, and non-exercising hip stationary. Hips and shoulders must remain square throughout exercise.

E. Push exercising leg back and gradually turn foot out slightly until gluteal is fully contracted. The exercising leg should end slightly out and away from midline of body.

F. Keep the chest up, rib cage lifted, bellybutton drawn toward spine and the lumbar spine in its neutral curvature.

G. Switch foot positions and repeat equal amounts of repetitions with other leg.

START

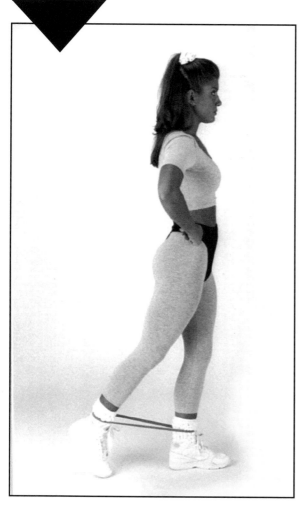

END

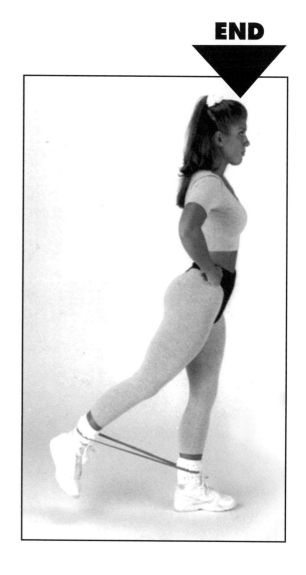

XERCISE BAND STANDING LEG CURL
(Hamstrings)

A. Place Xercise Band around both lower legs just above ankle height.

B. Stagger feet so foot of exercising leg is straight and slightly behind foot of non-exercising leg. Point toes of exercising leg down and keep them in contact with floor with heel up.

C. Place hands on hips or hold onto an object out in front of body at waist height if stabilization is too demanding.

D. Keep foot of non-exercising leg on floor, knee slightly bent, and non-exercising hip stationary. Hips and shoulders must remain square throughout exercise.

E. Flex knee and curl leg toward buttocks until hamstring is fully contracted.

F. Keep the chest up, rib cage lifted, bellybutton drawn toward spine and the lumbar spine in its neutral curvature.

G. Switch foot positions and repeat equal amounts of repetitions with other leg.

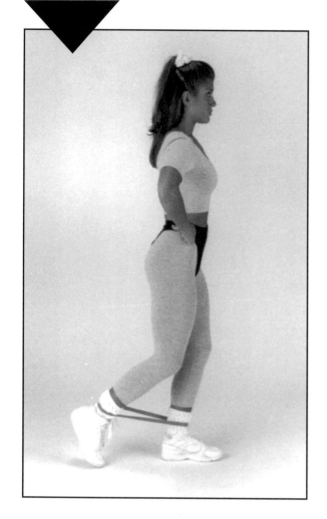

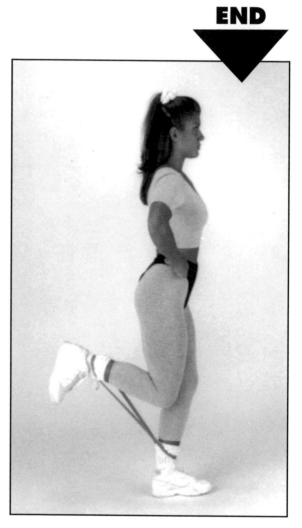

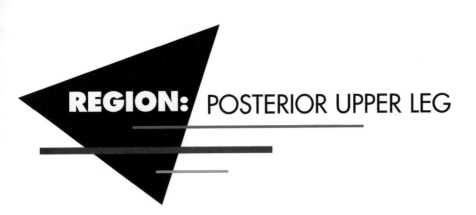

XERCISE BAND PRONE LEG CURL
(Hamstrings)

A. Place Xercise Band around both lower legs just above ankle height.

B. Lie on stomach, place back of hands under chin and extend both legs. Place a pador rolled up towel under knee of exercising leg for extra comfort if desired.

C. Pull toes of exercising foot toward shin to a neutral ankle position.

D. Keep hip bones in contact with floor, flex knee and curl leg toward buttocks until hamstring is fully contracted.

E. Repeat equal amounts of repetitions with other leg.

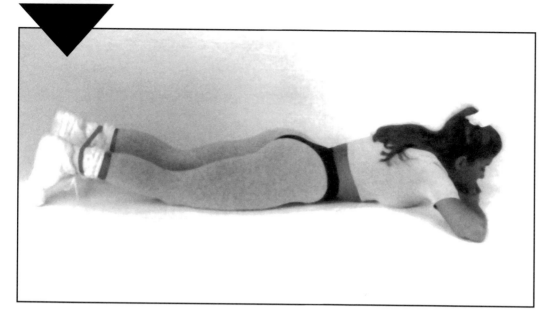

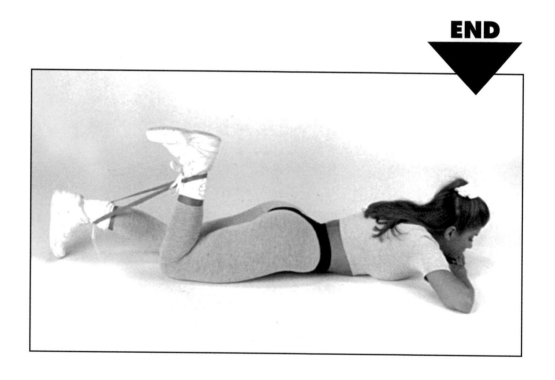

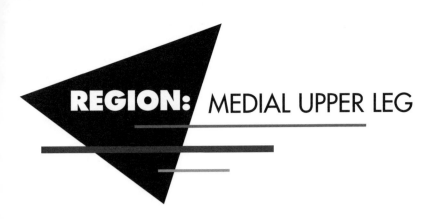

REGION: MEDIAL UPPER LEG

XERCISE BAND STANDING STRAIGHT/BENT LEG HIP ADDUCTION

(Adductors/Hip Internal Rotators)

A. From a standing position, place Xercise Band around exercising lower leg at calf height. If needed, place band higher toward knees to lessen resistance and decrease stress upon knee ligaments.

B. Have partner hold other end of Xercise Band taut or use attachable door strap and anchor at mid-calf height. Partner or attachment is positioned outside exercising leg.

C. Keep foot of non-exercising leg on floor, knee slightly bent and non-exercising hip stationary. Hips and shoulders must remain square throughout exercise.

D. With exercising leg fully abducted, place hands on hips or hold onto an object at side of body at waist height if stabilization is too demanding.

E. STRAIGHT LEG - Keep leg straight, lead with heel, pull forward and inward until adductors are fully contracted. End slightly in front of non-exercising foot. Do not allow knee of non-exercising leg to rotate.

BENT LEG - Lead with knee, drive it up and inward until adductors are fully contracted. End with heel in contact with inside of non-exercising knee.

F. Keep the chest up, rib cage lifted, bellybutton drawn toward spine and the lumbar spine in its neutral curvature.

G. Place the Xercise Band around the other lower leg and repeat equal amounts of repetitions.

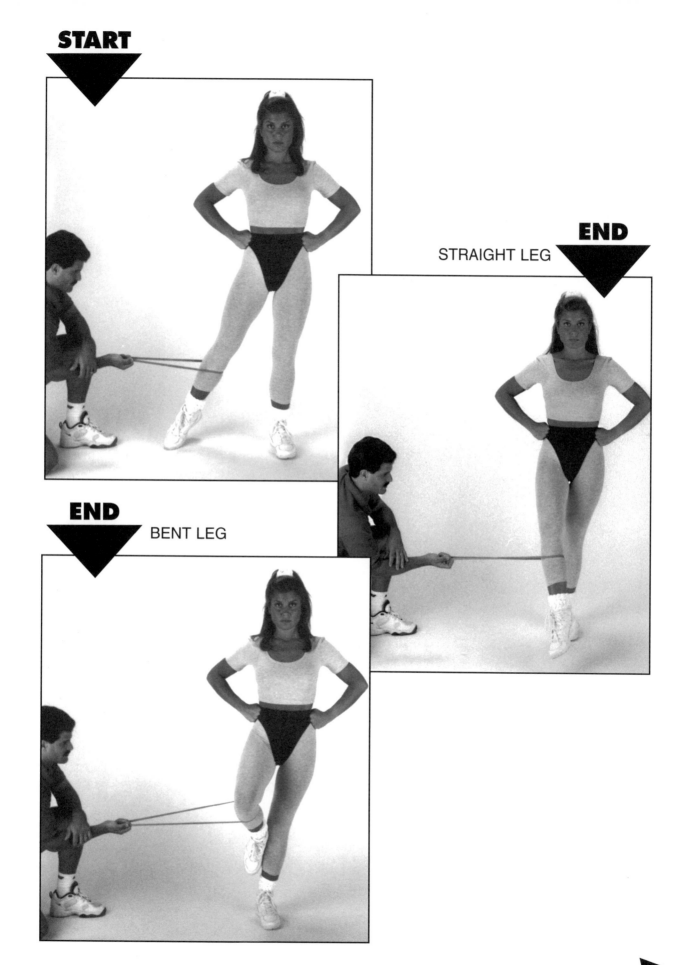

START

END
STRAIGHT LEG

END
BENT LEG

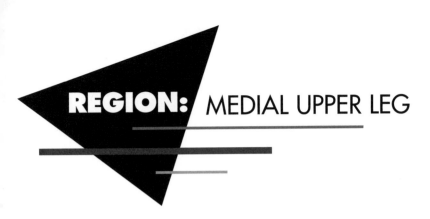

XERCISE BAND SEATED STRAIGHT LEG HIP ADDUCTION

(Adductors/Hip Internal Rotators)

▼ Position - Elbow or Hand Supported

A. From a seated position, place Xercise Band around exercising lower leg at calf height. If needed, place band higher toward knees to lessen resistance and decrease stress upon knee ligaments.

B. Have partner hold other end of Xercise Band taut or use attachable door strap and anchor at ankle height. Partner or attachment is positioned outside exercising leg.

C. With exercising leg fully abducted, lie back supporting upper body on elbows or with hands. The exercising leg should be straightened with hip rotated so toes point outward.

D. Keep leg straight, pull up and in toward bent knee while gradually rotating hip inward. End knee to knee, toes inward, and adductors fully contracted.

E. Keep the chest up, rib cage lifted, bellybutton drawn toward spine and the lumbar spine in its neutral curvature.

F. Place the Xercise Band around the other lower leg and repeat equal amounts of repetitions.

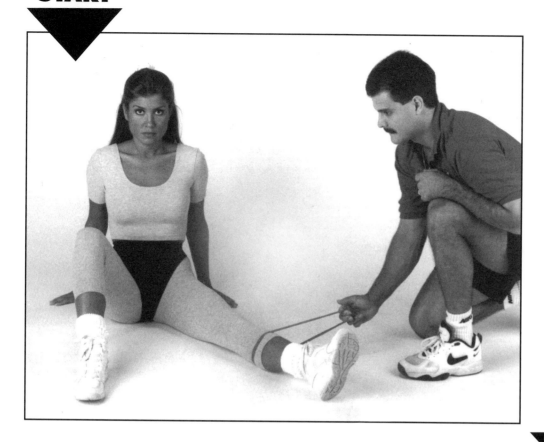

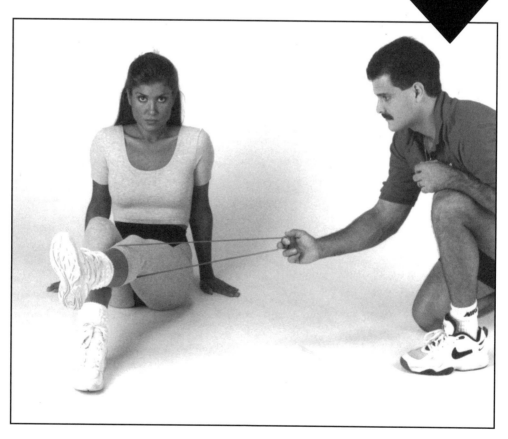

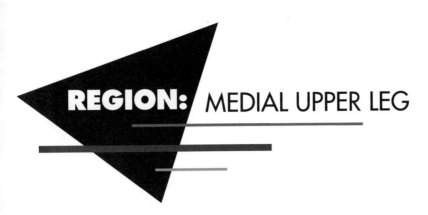

XERCISE BAND SIDE LYING STRAIGHT LEG HIP ADDUCTION

(Adductors)

A. From a seated position, bend non-exercising leg fully so heel is parallel to opposite knee. Place Xercise Band under arch of foot and point toes forward.

B. Place other end of Xercise Band at mid-calf height of exercising leg and straighten.

C. Lie on side and roll onto hip of exercising leg. Rotate hip outward so toes point away from body.

D. Bend arm and support body weight on elbow. Place other hand across body on floor to stabilize pelvis.

E. Keep leg straight, lead with heel and pull up and in toward bent knee until adductors are fully contracted. End with knees parallel to one another.

F. Keep the chest up, rib cage lifted, bellybutton drawn toward spine and the lumbar spine in its neutral curvature.

G. Roll onto other side, switch foot positions and repeat equal amounts of repetitions with other leg.

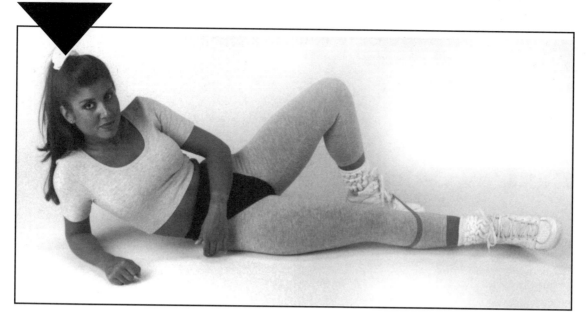

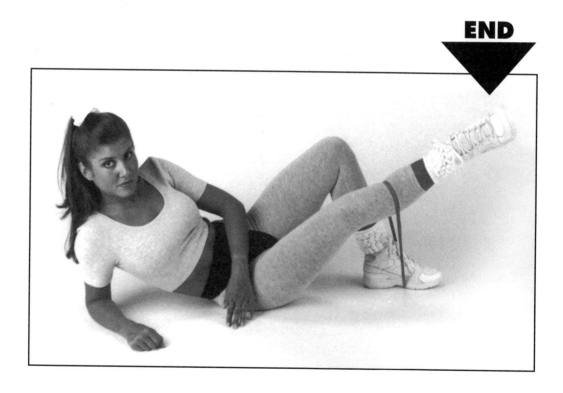

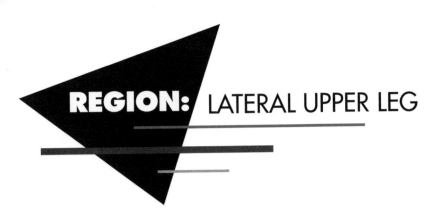

XERCISE BAND STANDING STRAIGHT LEG HIP ABDUCTION

(Abductors)

A. From a standing position, place Xercise Band around lower legs at calf height. If needed, place band higher toward knees to lessen resistance and decrease stress upon knee ligaments.

B. Place hands on hips or hold onto an object at side of body at waist height if stabilization is too demanding.

C. Rotate hip of exercising leg inward. Keep leg straight, lead with heel and push outward as far as possible. The opposite hip and shoulders must remain stationary.

D. Keep the chest up, rib cage lifted, bellybutton drawn toward spine and the lumbar spine in its neutral curvature.

E. Repeat equal amounts of repetitions with other leg.

This exercise may also be performed in a walking fashion by placing Xercise Band around both lower legs. The Xercise Band will need to be moved higher toward knee to maintain straight leg position. Use the same mechanics as in point C. Keep hands on hips and shoulders square while walking.

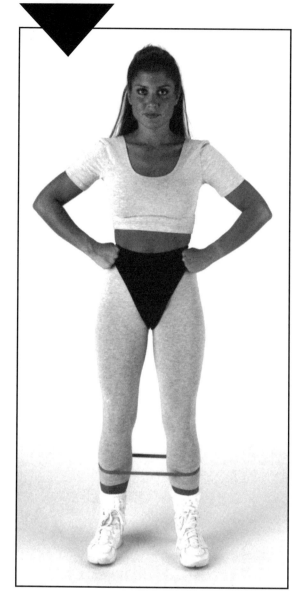

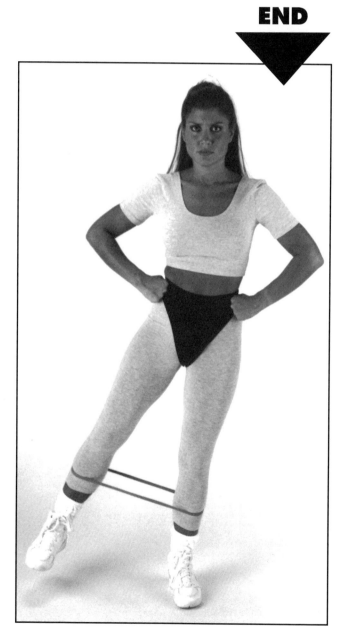

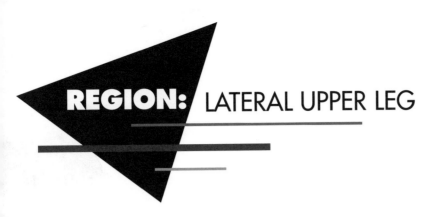

REGION: LATERAL UPPER LEG

XERCISE BAND SIDE LYING STRAIGHT LEG HIP ABDUCTION

(Abductors)

A. Sit and place Xercise Band around lower legs. If needed, place band higher toward knees to lessen resistance and decrease stress upon knee ligaments.

B. Lie on side and roll onto hip of non-exercising leg.

C. Bend arm that rests on floor overhead and place head on shoulder. Place other hand across body on floor to stabilize pelvis.

D. Extend both legs fully, lead with heel and push upward as high as possible. The opposite hip must remain stationary.

E. Keep the chest up, rib cage lifted, bellybutton drawn toward spine and the lumbar spine in its neutral curvature.

F. Roll onto other side and repeat equal amounts of repetitions with other leg.

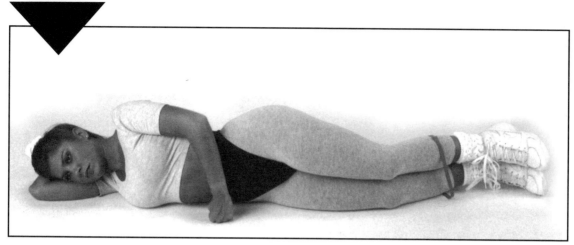

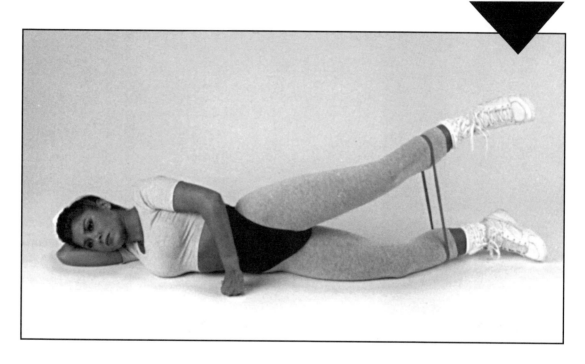

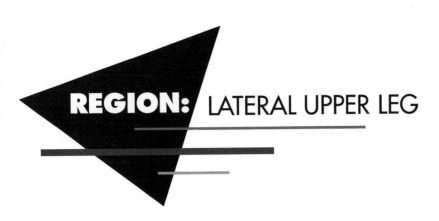

XERCISE BAND BACK LYING HIP ABDUCTION FROM FLEXED HIP POSITION

(Abductors)

A. Sit and place Xercise Band around lower legs at calf height. If needed, place band higher toward knees to lessen resistance and decrease stress upon knee ligaments.

B. Lie on back and place hands on floor next to hips.

C. Raise legs until arch is taken out of low back (flat back position). Legs may be in a slightly bent position.

D. Point toes inward, lead with heels and push outward as far as possible. The back must remain in its flat back position.

E. Keep the chest up, rib cage lifted, bellybutton drawn toward spine and the lumbar spine in its neutral curvature.

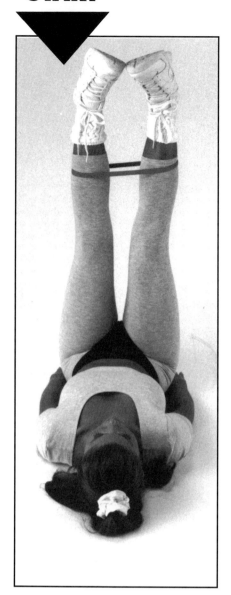

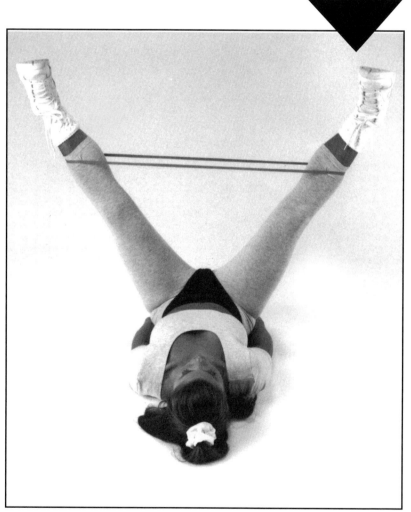

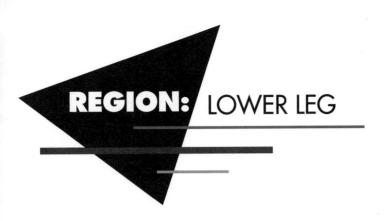

XERCISE BAND SEATED ANKLE PLANTAR FLEXION

(Ankle Plantar Flexors)

A. Sit on floor or elevated platform with exercising leg straight and non-exercising leg fully bent with heel slightly forward of knee with foot flat.

B. Grasp one end of Xercise Band with both hands and place other end around ball of straight leg foot.

C. Raise heel off floor, or position over edge of elevated platform keeping thighs stationary, and press toes downward against Xercise Band as far as possible (plantar flexion).

D. Contraction should be felt in back of lower leg.

E. Keep the chest up, rib cage lifted, bellybutton drawn toward spine and the lumbar spine in its neutral curvature.

F. Switch foot positions and repeat equal amounts of repetitions with other leg.

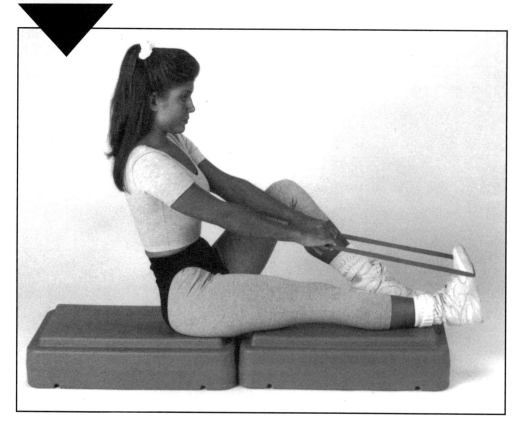

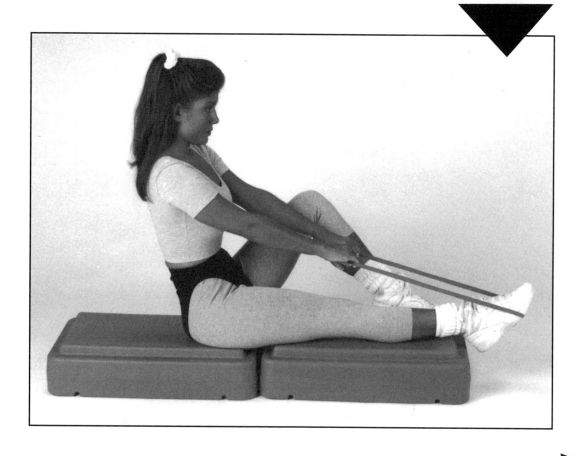

THE COMPLETE GUIDE TO **RUBBERIZED RESISTANCE EXERCISES** 347

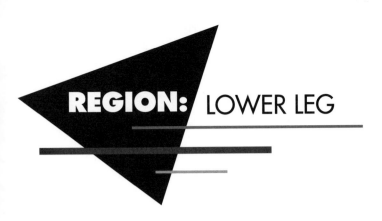

XERCISE BAND SEATED ANKLE EVERSION (Dual)

(Ankle Evertors)

A. Sit on floor and place Xercise Band around forefoot of both feet. Place hands under shoulders.

B. Separate legs as far as needed for proper tension and point toes inward.

C. Keep thighs stationary and push little toes outward as far as possible (eversion).

D. Contraction should be felt in outer portion of ankle and lower leg.

E. Keep the chest up, rib cage lifted, bellybutton drawn toward spine and the lumbar spine in its neutral curvature.

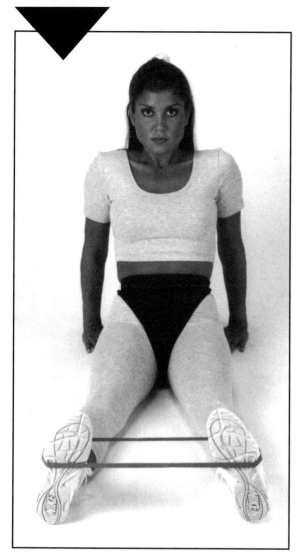

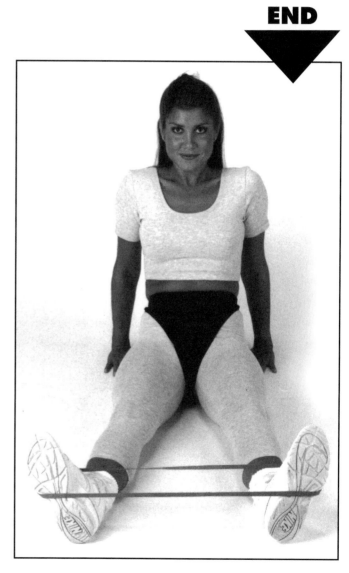

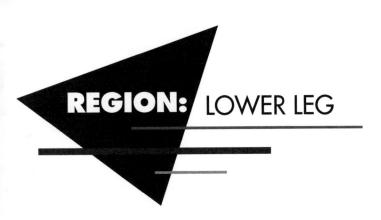

REGION: LOWER LEG

XERCISE BAND SEATED ANKLE INVERSION
(Ankle Invertors)

A. Sit on bench or elevated platform with ankles just over edge when using partner. Sit on floor and place pad or rolled up towel under calf of exercising leg if using attachable doorstop.

B. Place Xercise Band around exercising forefoot. Have partner hold other end of Xercise Band taut or use attachable door strap and anchor at ankle height. Partner should place hand on exercising lower leg to stabilize hip. Partner or attachment is positioned outside exercising leg.

C. Rotate foot of exercising leg outward (eversion). Keep thigh stationary and pull big toe inward as far as possible (inversion).

D. Contraction should be felt in inner portion of ankle and lower leg.

E. Keep the chest up, rib cage lifted, bellybutton drawn toward spine and the lumbar spine in its neutral curvature.

F. Place the Xercise Band around the other forefoot and repeat equal amounts of repetitions.

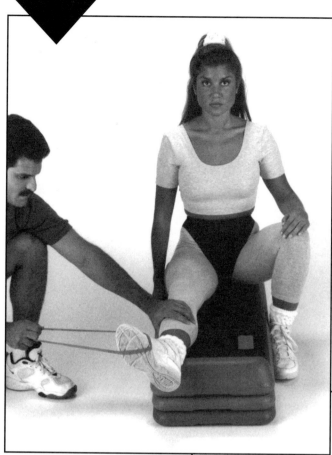

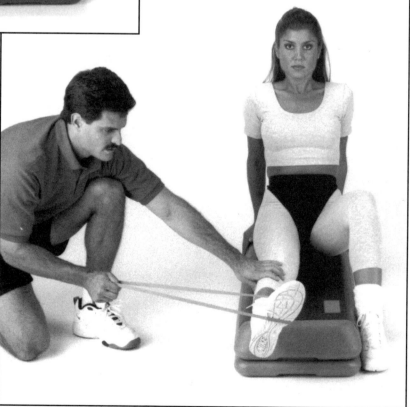

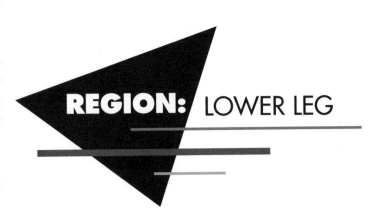

REGION: LOWER LEG

XERCISE BAND SEATED ANKLE DORSI FLEXION (Dual)

(Ankle Dorsiflexors)

A. Sit on bench or elevated platform with ankles just over edge or sit on floor and place pad or rolled up towel under calves. Position hands under shoulders and grasp outside of bench.

B. Bend knees slightly and place Xercise Bands around forefoot and have partner hold Xercise Bands taut. Partner is positioned in front of lower legs.

C. Keep thighs stationary and pull toes toward shins as far as possible (dorsi flexion).

D. Contraction should be felt in front lower leg.

E. Keep the chest up, rib cage lifted, bellybutton drawn toward spine and the lumbar spine in its neutral curvature.

> **TECH TIPS**
> **This exercise may be performed unilaterally.**

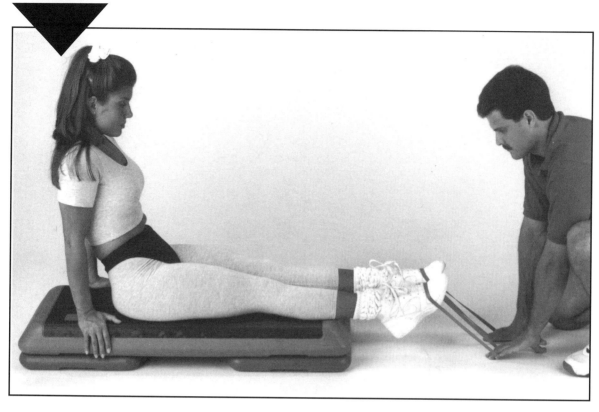

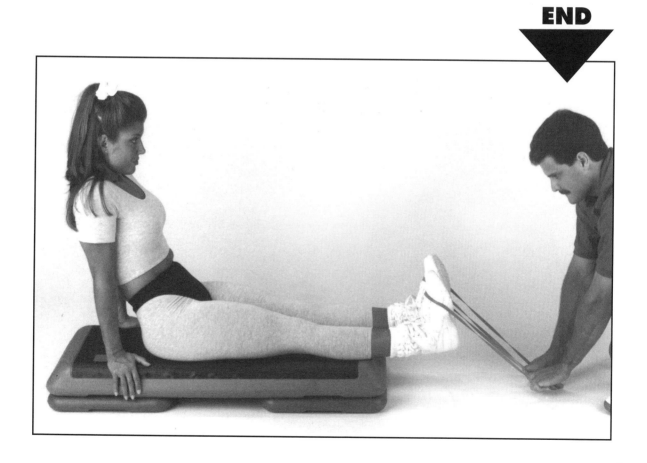